THE MIDLIFE
CYCLIST

THE MIDLIFE
CYCLIST

THE ROAD MAP FOR THE +40 RIDER
WHO WANTS TO TRAIN HARD,
RIDE FAST AND STAY HEALTHY

PHIL CAVELL

BLOOMSBURY SPORT
LONDON • OXFORD • NEW YORK • NEW DELHI • SYDNEY

BLOOMSBURY SPORT
Bloomsbury Publishing Plc
50 Bedford Square, London, WC1B 3DP, UK
29 Earlsfort Terrace, Dublin 2, Ireland

BLOOMSBURY, BLOOMSBURY SPORT and the Diana logo are trademarks of
Bloomsbury Publishing Plc

First published in Great Britain 2021

A catalogue record for this book is available from the British Library

Library of Congress Cataloguing-in-Publication data has been applied for

ISBN: TPB: 978-1-4729-6138-9; eBook: 978-1-4729-6139-6

10 9

Typeset in Adobe Garamond Pro by Deanta Global Publishing Services, Chennai, India
Printed and bound in Great Britain by CPI Group (UK) Ltd. Croydon, CR0 4YY

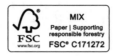

To find out more about our authors and books visit www.bloomsbury.com
and sign up for our newsletters

CONTENTS

PROLOGUE

One Saturday, almost a quarter of a century ago, I raced at the Eastway criterium circuit in East London. It was a grander event than local riders like me generally got the opportunity to ride in. That meant competing against better riders from all over the UK, as well as a smattering of Team Telecom Academy riders, in their distinctive pink jerseys, from Germany. I forget how I even wangled an entry. I remember better London-based riders than me turning up to spectate and even 'congratulating' me on having the confidence to line up in such company. Brian Fleming came and shook hands with me and wished me luck. We both knew what he meant. Brian was a local star and one of the best bunch sprinters in South East England at the time. Brian was warm, generous and sincere off the circuit, but a caged fighter in the heat of criterium combat. I liked him immensely and was very pleased to see him, but also faintly alarmed that a rider of his calibre was not racing himself.

Eastway was the most dynamic and majestic criterium circuit ever devised. I think even Eddy Merckx agreed with that sentiment after racing there in 1977 (he lost to Sid Barrass). Uniquely, Eastway's topographical variance and tight corners had the capacity to reward every facet of a rider's arsenal – technical skill, explosive power, endurance and mental fortitude. A million ways to test yourself and your competition – a cathedral of pain. I loved Eastway beyond reason.

The race was 50 miles – 50 one-mile laps. Fifty times up Oxo Hill, 50 times around Claries Hairpin – leaning over so far that it felt like your knee would brush the tarmac (I still have the scars from the times that became a reality) – and 50 times up the false flat, eastwards into a headwind, past the start–finish line, clubhouse and spectators.

London riders always wanted to race out of their skins on home turf, especially against really tough competition. That is the moment that passed between Brian and me and what I felt when the race unusually exploded on the first lap. No gentle probing exploration and sideways glances or strategic line-outs by the stronger teams. The race detonated anaerobically, and somewhat irrationally, for the first few laps. As a veteran local rider I was one of the fastest around Claries Hairpin, which preceded Oxo Hill. This put me into the middle of an almost full-throttle bunch sprint in 53-12 up the steepest 1-in-10 section of the climb. When I looked back from the top of the hill I could see something every road racer lives for – a useful amount of clean air to the chasing peloton. Only this time it was myself and seven other vastly superior riders comprising an eight-man break. Over the next 20 laps we went through metronomically until we had a half-a-lap gap to the bunch. As I remember, the only other 'London' rider in the break was Garry Baker (but I don't trust my memory in this instance for reasons that will become clear). It's usual during a long breakaway for weaker riders to miss a pull at the front, or at least try to soft-pedal through their turn. Pride precluded the former, and the speed of every rider in the break the latter. It took all my strength just to go over the top of the rider in front of me, to the point that I was looking for the second weakest rider in the breakaway to see if I could cut in the line behind them, to make my own through and off movements easier. But there was no second weakest rider.

The inevitable circadian rhythm of the break meant that my turn at the front seemed to occur just as we went up the invisible hill, into the wind, across the start–finish line. But still a cocktail of pride and stubbornness prevailed over my body's pain and inclination to stop. My conscious brain imprinted itself over all my natural physical pain reflexes, right up to the point when it couldn't. Then I passed out on the bike in front of the assembled spectators at the start–finish area, and ploughed straight off the track and into the chain-link fence in front of Eastway's iconic clubhouse.

I was out for only a few seconds. The first thing I saw was Brian bending over me and checking I was unhurt, beyond my injured pride. I was fine – I had simply stretched my physical envelope too far and had made too good a friend of pain. But the fundamentals were that I was young, fit, strong and largely conditioned for the exertions I had placed upon my body. The operative term for the purpose of this book is, of course, 'young'.

Would I push myself to that brink of physical shutdown, either in training or competition, at my current age of 58? That's the main question behind this book. If the answer is 'no', then where is the line that I will not cross and what is its intellectual underpinning? If the answer is 'yes', and I should push the performance envelope without regard to age, then am I risking injury or even death?

There may well have been plenty of times when our human ancestors pushed themselves to the brink of physical collapse, fleeing predators or pursuing food. But until very recently, the chances of someone surviving to even 40 years old were vanishingly rare. Indeed, the life expectancy of pre-industrial humans was about 30 years, so for all but a handful of our 300,000 generations of evolution from the great ape, a 40-year-old human is genetically irrelevant, a selective aberration.

Nature is, in that sense, crushingly indifferent as to whether a 40-year-old ancestor outruns a predator or shakes off an infected cut. There was simply no genetic imperative for early humans to survive into middle age and beyond. To use a term that would infuriate evolutionary biologists – we're existing outside of our 'design life'. The lifespan of the tiny number of humans who managed to live into old age was of no consequence on a genetic level. They would have either bred and raised their young by the age of 40, or missed their opportunity. Beyond being a sinewy snack for a passing predator, nature is blind to the event of their deaths.

Irrelevant – but not necessarily redundant

A 30-year lifespan seemed to be the upper end of the age spectrum for hundreds of thousands of generations of our ancestors for a very good reason. It allowed the individual to mature, breed and parent offspring to maturity. So, while there's certainly evolutionary pressure for Homo sapiens to survive to 30 years old, that still leaves me very unlikely to win an all-out sprint against my 29-year-old self, whether on a bicycle at Eastway or running away from a hungry leopard. I'll almost certainly lose because there's plainly no selective imperative for me to win. Indeed, if you take a strictly gene-centric view, there's actually a selective advantage to me losing a sprint for survival against a younger close family member, so they can survive and propagate shared genes through their offspring.

Remember that we're genetically almost identical to our modern human ancestors from tens of thousands of years ago. It's true that the process of evolution is continual, but it's also true that there has been simply too little time and too few generations for substantive changes to the human genome.

But this shouldn't lead us to think that we're redundant just because our genomes didn't evolve to last past our late 20s. Paleoanthropologist Rachel Caspari points to an exponential boost in art, culture and civic activity in the Upper Paleolithic era 30,000 years ago, at the same time as a demographic deflection or a shift in lifespan took place, resulting in our ancestors actually living long enough to become invested and contributing grandparents. Initially, Caspari was unsure whether the lifespan uplift in adult survivorship was due to biological/genetic factors or behavioural shifts. After screening our older ancestors from the Middle Paleolithic era – between 140,000 and 40,000 years ago – it became clear that a cultural shift had helped Stone Age grandparents make their offsprings' lives markedly less Hobbesian – i.e. 'nasty, brutish and short'.

Performance pioneers

We're almost certainly the first cohort, in a great enough number, to be statistically relevant, to push our bodies into and beyond middle age, towards peak performance. We're the virtual crash-test dummies for future generations who refuse to succumb to evolutionary stereotyping. How many of our parents were interested in structured training for the sake of pure performance, past the age of 40 or 50? So, nobody really knows for sure what happens if you try to tune your engine to racing performance, at an age when at any other time in history you would have been dead for years if not decades. This is a critical time and we're the pathfinder generation for those that follow us.

Spooling back to Eastway 25 years ago, I rode the few miles home reflecting that at least I knew where the line was. I raced the next day and pushed myself almost as hard.

INTRODUCTION

Currently, there's a quiet revolution occurring in the ranks of middle-aged and older sportsmen and women. Virtually nothing happened in several hundred thousand generations, in terms of mass participation of veteran athletes in structured training, and now for the first time, in the space of just two generations, we are seeing a fitness surge at scale. Most of our parents and grandparents wouldn't have participated in hard training post-marriage and certainly not after the birth of their first child, as soccer and netball were inevitably replaced with fondue parties and trips to the pub. At the very most, our parents may just have embraced (probably way too late) the '70s and '80s keep-fit crazes – jogging or aerobics. As our middle-aged generation ages, we've decided to plant our flag on the more distant but brighter star of elite performance, achieved through the application of quasi-professional sports science and technology.

The weapon of choice for this new genus of veteran athlete is often the bicycle. There are many reasons for this (which we will explore in this book) – cycling is generally gentle on ageing joints, every ride carries a sense of adventure, it's innately sociable and there are lots of measurable metrics. The preferred playgrounds are very varied, too – anywhere from epic Tour de France stages and days in the Serra de Tramuntana mountain ranges in Mallorca, to the now iconic Box Hill in Surrey or even Zwift(ing) in your own spare room.

I remember training camps in Mallorca 25 years ago. We were attracted by the promise of early season good weather (although Mallorca's 'Emerald Isle' nickname does more than hint at its precipitative nature) as well as the epic scenery and an overall feeling of quiet and space. Mallorca a quarter of a century ago was a yet-to-be-discovered fantasy playground for cyclists, and consequently many of the routes included unpaved roads that only added to the drama. The only tourist traffic seemed to be vintage car rallies that were often even slower up the Sa Colobra climb than we were. Now every road has been sealed and polished to within an inch of its life, as the government has realised that cyclists make exceptional tourists – we travel light, eat out a lot, don't pollute, generally don't get in trouble, and stop for copious amounts of strong coffee and Ensaïmada Mallorquina sweet bread.

In 25 years, or one short generation, Mallorca has shifted from a quiet training location for the few, and package holiday destination for the many, to a virtual Sims Island dedicated to the art of performance biking, for the new generation of riders. It is a microcosm of how cycling has shifted the centre of gravity of mass-participation sport.

As veteran athletes, we're completely unique in evolutionary terms – around 6.3 million adults are using cycling for sport and leisure in the UK – with a particularly steep increase in the number of female cyclists. Nevertheless, relatively little is known about what happens when you race-tune the engine of a 50- or 60-year-old to as close to Olympic levels as is currently humanly and scientifically possible. As the clinicians and sports scientists scrabble to catch up with newly commissioned research and data, this exponentially expanding group of women and men relentlessly push themselves further away from the shadow of generations before them, and towards the performance levels associated with professional athletes. I have clients in their late 50s (and even early 60s) who can ride at an average of 50km/h for 16km or more. This requires sustained power outputs significantly north of 300 watts (depending on the individual's aero efficiency), which is over double the level produced by an average untrained 20-year-old.

But just because we can, does that mean we necessarily should? Using contributions from cardiologists, pro-team physicians, coaches and nutritionists, this book evaluates the newest research, and where that research is missing, adds informed opinion, to formulate the gold-standard paradigm for the midlife cyclist, who wants to ride fast but also live long and stay healthy.

It is an almost universal truism that cycling is addictive. It combines, speed, fitness, adventure and adrenaline; but it's also uniquely functional and practical. There's something appealing about the prospect of waking up early in London and knowing that it's entirely within your current capability to ride to Devon in time for tea. It combines endurance, strength, agility, coordination and mental toughness. Imagine it's started to rain, the temperature is dropping, you're out of food and Exeter is still 30km away – do you stick or twist? The answer is, of course, that you twist.

I have a client called Ray, who is a decade into a burgeoning cycling career, at 60 years of age. Ray has gradually increased his fitness and mileage, to the point where he thinks nothing of getting the train to Penzance in Cornwall, then riding non-stop to Land's End and back to London, a distance of nearly 500km. I sometimes get an email from a Cornish lane or Wiltshire plain, with a picture of his custom Seven bike parked up while Ray takes in a pasty and a bottle of Coke. Ray is physically and mentally one of the fittest 60-year-olds on the planet (and, by the way, looks no more than 45). He relates his travels with such passion, and is constantly planning his next adventure to push himself even harder. He recently finished the epic Paris–Brest–Paris very close to the front. It's fair to say that Ray has become addicted – there are worse addictions to have.

Pushing ourselves physically as we age is almost certainly mostly positive, as well as fun, which we shall see going through this book. But we need to be mindful of the risks and pitfalls, one of which is falling off. If you ride a bike, just as if you ride a horse, there's always a chance that you could have a tumble. You can mitigate the risk by improving your technical riding skills, not riding in the ice and snow, making sure your riding position is optimised, and ensuring that your bike is fit for purpose and regularly serviced. But the fact remains – the more you ride, the greater your chances of eventually falling. If you do fall off, your injuries will often be no worse than a moment of embarrassment or cuts and bruises. If the fall is a little more serious, then collarbones, hips and wrists are likely candidates for trauma. Up the ante, and pelvises and backs may suffer. But in 20 years, we at Cyclefit have very rarely seen an injury from which a rider has not been able to fully recover. Or as Dr Nigel Stephens so eloquently frames the proposition: 'As cyclists, we trade hugely improved cardiovascular and cognitive health for occasional orthopaedic trauma.' (Stephens is a consultant cardiologist, European Masters Champion and midlife cyclist, and we'll meet him again later.)

But as we age our tolerance for error or injury inevitably reduces – throwing youth at any physical problem is normally the most successful strategy. But when you no longer have access to the elixir of youth, the next best strategy is being well informed about every aspect of your riding practice.

The problems we commonly see, outside of an accident-induced trauma, are generally caused by an information and moderation deficit. For example, foot pain arises because an athlete's shoe wasn't chosen to suit their foot type, or there's an incorrectly aligned cleat-pedal interface. Or back, neck and shoulder pain appears due to incorrect positioning and posture on the bike. Knee injuries, while not as prevalent as they are for runners, are still common. The knee is a big hinge joint in the middle of the leg and can only tolerate misalignment for so long before pain sets in. If a problem is tackled early, or during its acute phase, removal of the underlying cause is enough to instantly deal with the pain, and the problem goes away. If a rider ignores an issue it's likely to become chronic – the affected tissues and structures are now damaged.

Removal of the underlying cause (change of shoe, pedal cleat or bike position) won't be enough and physical therapy will likely be needed to fix the affected area. Ergo – as a veteran athlete, don't allow problems to become chronic!

This book also looks at whether research and guidance is different for midlife women and midlife men (spoiler alert – it is), and how that may be differently expressed in our training and racing instincts. Do men have a lot to learn from women in this regard? (Second spoiler alert – they probably do.) We want to help both sexes to ride fast and live long.

We start the book with rather humbling first principles – that reaching middle age at all is a formidable achievement, as we've seen already. In a quarter of a million years we have wandered and now cycled the planet, but it is only in the last century that getting past 40 years of age has been a real possibility. And as a possible consequence, how the veteran human form reacts to being physically pushed to the extreme is still fairly poorly understood. Bluntly, in evolutionary terms we are not really meant to be alive at all, and almost certainly would not be at any other time in history. The experts and doctors in part hypothesise, speculate and theorise about how the ageing body reacts to high performance. Their frustration at not having all the answers at their fingertips is palpable and provides the impetus for much of their current research and thinking.

The book then takes you on a magical biological tour of your ageing body, to understand what's happening at a cellular level as we all get older. It looks at how exercise (especially cycling) can be used as a panacea for solving the worst physical and cognitive effects of ageing as an athlete. It's something I've heard time and again from the medical community (people not normally given to hyperbole) – no drug or medical intervention has ever been devised that has the efficacy and power of simple movement, at any age.

You can't have a midlife cyclist without having a bicycle. We take the opportunity to study this wonderful machine that we all seem to venerate unquestioningly. We also examine the first principles surrounding these miraculous machines – how did the bike evolve in the first place? Is it still the best expression of human biomechanics, over 130 years since it was first invented? Is the bicycle really humanity's finest ever invention? Or have we just neglected to rethink the basics? We use our decades as cycling biomechanists to critically review how well the bicycle expresses our human potential, and why the basic bicycle architecture has remained valid, but largely stagnant, for so long.

We also consider the big questions surrounding cycling as a fitness tool – is it fundamentally different to other forms of exercise? And, just as importantly, is cycling all you should do to stay fit and healthy or should you be supplementing cycling with doses of other exercise? (Another spoiler – you should.)

Which leads us onto the most important question of all in 'Will I Die?' Will doing more of what you love, kill you or make you better? The press loves to run poorly researched, sensational articles about how intense exercise could hurt or even kill you, should you exercise hard into middle age. They are cynically exploiting a temporary knowledge gap to sell their newspapers and magazines. We consult with world-leading cardiologists and cyclists, and review the latest research for a calmer, deeper assessment of the likely outcome of riding as hard as you like as you get older. And whether outcomes may differ for men and women.

Let's be very clear from the start – this book isn't a training manual. There are many fabulous books that will walk you through periodised training methods, but this book explores the concept and philosophy of training, and whether it applies differently to midlife athletes. We question the underlying principles of training for cycling in 'Midlife Performance – Too Late for Speed?'

In 'Food for Sport', we ponder how our nutritional requirements alter as we get older, but as we still endeavour to exercise at the highest level possible. We also review how we might change our dietary strategies to both maximise performance and maintain long-term health.

The 'Bikes, Bike Fit and Biomechanics' chapter is our professional happy place, and is how we've spent almost every working day for the last 20 years, working at Cyclefit, helping professional and amateur athletes and teams of all ages and aspiration. We've also taught bike fitting all around the world to a new generation of student technicians, who are keen to help their own clients function better on their bikes. We've jammed every secret and nugget of information that we've ever gleaned about how folk interact with their bikes into this chapter. It is truly our greatest hits section.

The final chapter, 'The Mindful Cyclist', gathered importance during the writing of the book. It grew from a single sentence into an entire chapter. Why? Because every consultant, medic, coach and athlete that we interviewed went out of their way to highlight the emerging importance of a holistic mind-body approach to effectively balancing hard training, ageing and general life health. All the cardiologists flagged up unspecified 'inflammation' as a possible contributor to potential problems. We look in depth at the role of the autonomic nervous system, alcohol and even sleep to help you become faster, calmer and healthier.

Mindfulness is almost certainly where the gold is buried in terms of harmonising future performance and longevity for any athlete, but most especially midlife cyclists. Our contention is that professional teams will spend ever more resources and time in this arena, as a way of achieving and preserving athlete performance.

The Midlife Cyclist has, in truth, been in gestation for many years, but was substantially written during the Covid-19 pandemic, which will hopefully seem less devastating and frightening at the time of reading than it was at the time of writing. There will be many dire consequences of this destructive disease, but one of the positive outcomes may well be that more people are choosing bikes for both fitness and transport. Covid-19 has also bought into focus two potential fault lines that fall within the scope of this book. The first is that the potentially more deleterious outcomes of the disease appear to fall disproportionally on older age groups, which seems to suggest that middle-aged people and older aren't just young people who grew up and got old, but are fundamentally changed because of the ageing process. Which isn't at all how living with advancing age feels, since when we look in the mirror every morning, we feel largely the same as we did yesterday, last week or even last year. Covid-19 has shown us that this is a misguided and simplistic supposition, and that we're actually profoundly and structurally different at 55 than we were at 25, and as a consequence, the risk from Covid-19 seems to increase exponentially as we age. Secondly, the incidence of Covid-19 appears to have demonstrated that higher levels of aerobic fitness can protect against the damaging effects of the disease in older age groups, possibly by strengthening the immune system and mediating its response to the disease.

The complex and highly interactive relationship between age, health and athletic fitness is the holy triumvirate – there are many out there who feel that only two can increase significantly at any one time – age and fitness or age and health.

We ran the Midlife Cyclist Lecture Series in 2017 and 2018 at the Cyclefit store in Covent Garden, London. We had wonderful, warm and generous speakers who contributed for free in the spirit of joint exploration and education – many are featured elsewhere in this book. The lecture slots filled up as soon as they were launched online and then we let people in so they could listen and ask questions.

Men, women, mums, dads, grandparents and concerned grown-up children all in search of enlightenment on that key question – can we use the bicycle to simultaneously get fitter and healthier as we get older? Indeed, it's the humble aim of this book to square that troublesome triangle.

Phil Cavell, 2020

1

THE AGEING CYCLIST – GROWING OLD DISGRACEFULLY

The conscious part of me wants to exercise because it's good for me – the benefits are proven, uncontroversial and listed in various forms in nearly every chapter of this book. I'm also fairly sure that I'm compelled to exercise unrestrainedly and push myself physically as an unconscious death-avoidance strategy. I'm trying to pedal or run away from the inexorable pull of an unyielding rope that's attached to all of us and extends an unknown distance across into the horizon. Getting old and dying is as much a part of our psychological DNA as it is our physical DNA – kids are aware of dying from a young age and talk about it openly. Their natural inquisitiveness is ameliorated by the fact that it tends to happen around them to fragile animals and elderly relatives.

If I sit quietly and think about it, I'm not even sure that I'm trying to avoid getting old and dying, as much as meeting it on my own terms. Harvard cell biologist Derick Rossi clinically captures this feeling perfectly: 'The [therapeutic] goal would be to increase health span, not lifespan.'

Substitute 'exercise' for 'therapeutic' and that could be my ethos captured in one very short sentence. Change the terms of engagement by continuing to train into middle age and beyond – lean in on exercise as the panacea to adaptively change my body for the better; to load the dice in favour of better, not necessarily more.

Ageing is scientifically one of the least understood areas of human health. Is that possibly because scientists are also human and therefore have a cognitive bias towards the holy grail of arresting, or even reversing, ageing instead of explaining the mechanisms at work?

Essentially we age at a cellular level – cataracts, cancers and arthritis all have a link to incremental imperfections in the way that DNA is repaired in our bodies as we age. We simply seem to get worse at copying ourselves as we get older – keep photocopying a picture of a daffodil, and inevitably across several generations the image will depower and smudge to something that barely resembles the original daffodil anymore. This process is called senescence – the progressive deterioration and loss of acuity as something tends towards death. We also know that as we get older DNA repair is increasingly less reliable, just as the daffodil gets gradually greyer and less distinct, but we still don't know why or how to arrest or reverse the process. But it's increasingly clear that exercise appears to be one of the most powerful positive interventions that we can make to affect ageing at a cellular level – and endurance running or cycling are best. Science is still trying to provide an explanation of the physiological mechanisms at play when midlife athletes push themselves in training and competition; however, increasing attention is being focussed on strands at the very end of our DNA, called telomeres.

The telomere story

The telomere story is actually quite exciting from the perspective of the midlife cyclist. The telomere is like a protective presta valve cap at the end of each strand of DNA – every time the cell divides, the telomere protects the chromosome. A chromosome is a strand of DNA inside the nucleus of our cells, which is imprinted with our genetic code. As humans we have 22 pairs of chomosomes plus one pair of XX or XY (female,

male) sex chromosomes, making 46 in total. However cell division appears to occur at the expense of a fractional shortening of the telomere itself. If the telomere becomes too short the cell risks moving into a senescence phase, which in turn affects organ function and lifespan. Some scientists have even suggested the telomere has a 'canary in the coal mine' role, and may be able to warn about potential issues, such as cancer. If telomeres are actually our genetic fuses smouldering deep inside our cells, the burning question has to be – is there a way to help them recover some of their former length? A recent German study, headed by Christian Werner, compared 124 people between the ages of 30 to 60 by subjecting them to four different exercise protocols: sedentary, high intensity (HIT), resistance (weight) training, and endurance. The result was that only endurance training and, to a degree, interval training (for example, hill repeats) had a tangible and beneficial effect on the length and function of the telomere: 'Endurance training and interval training, but not resistance training, increased telomerase activity and telomere length, which are important for cellular senescence, regenerative capacity, and thus, healthy ageing.'

Werner went on to suggest that the results could make sense from an evolutionary perspective – in the ancestral environment we needed to travel long distances as well as exhibit strong fight and flight reactions. This makes sense to me – from the perspective of this book, everything, always, must cogently link back to our evolved function, not what we now typically demand from our bodies in the modern world. We evolved to persistence hunt, not to sit and browse the internet; and endurance cycling obviously more closely mimics persistence hunting than playing video games.

Other studies seem to have confirmed Werner's findings, that exercise seems to change us on a cellular level by increasing the length of the protective cap at the end of our DNA strands. This is a huge epiphany if it continues to be corroborated by future research, as it means that increasing the amount of cycling we do can positively change us at a cellular level. Right now, I'm happy to believe that it's true.

Let's go back to my metaphor of the unyielding rope extending an unknown distance over the horizon, with its inexorable pull on our mortal existence – exercise alone may not be able to sever the rope completely, but it seems it can make it more elastic, buying us both time and better functionality.

Ageing happens at a cellular – or 'micro' – level, but we experience it on a zoomed-out 'macro' level, which expresses itself in how we look, feel and perform. And just as the right type and dosing of exercise provides a positive stimulus at a cellular level by increasing telomere length, it can also effect positive change at a macro level, all around our body. It's the primary object of this book to effectively calibrate all of the contributory factors that can positively influence cell health and ageing on a micro-level, and how you perform in the world on a bike at a macro level.

The midlife muscular-skeletal system

Let's make a general rule. Wherever possible I'll try to get the bad news out of the way first – I'm an eternal optimist and it fundamentally suits my personality to work like this. So the bad news is that we lose muscle fibres as we get older and can't grow new ones, unlike white blood cells, hair or nails. Although not completely understood, this muscle loss is well documented and has a name – sarcopenia, or age-related skeletal muscle atrophy. Sarcopenia is actually the loss of individual muscle fibres, which by attrition results in a very significant loss of muscle bulk – up to 50 per cent between the ages of 25 and 80 if you're a man, and generally less if you're a woman. The loss of three-dimensional muscle bulk is partly due to the declining number of our actual muscle fibres, but is also thought to be the result of changes to lifestyle and diet, as well as incremental neuromuscular transformations. On a chemical level, it's assumed that declining anabolic (anabolic means 'building up') hormone levels speed up the decrease in both the size and strength of our muscles.

That means that even if you exercise at the same level and have the same diet between the ages of 30 and 55, you'll still attritionally lose muscle size and strength. So, sarcopenia is something that we all need to understand and ameliorate whether we're athletes or not – and this is especially true for men. Moreover, sarcopenia seems to affect our Type II 'fast-twitch' power muscles more than our endurance-based Type I muscle fibres. This is a predictable, if not fully understood, pathogenesis (mechanism of disease). Losing muscle bulk and strength as we get older has inevitable performance consequences, but in an increasingly ageing population, has an even more profound public health significance. The average 80-year-old male uses 100 per cent of their muscular strength to stand up from a chair; hence it only takes a week sitting around because of illness or a fall to weaken to the point where that man cannot get up at all, which is thought to cause a cascade of other health issues. The inevitable conclusion has to be to commit to not being an average 80-year-old, and that starts with not being an average 50-year-old.

However, the extremely good news is that losing muscle bulk and strength isn't at all inevitable if we understand its pathology and are willing to push back hard against the time's arrow direction of travel. The route out of sarcopenia is highly directed resistance (weight) training, post 50 years of age. The only other route out is highly directed resistance training aided by performance-enhancing drugs – I wouldn't especially advise the latter because of the serious health risks, especially as we get older. So that just leaves hard work, then – which at our age we should already be used to. Targeted weight training will cause the muscle fibres that remain to hypertrophy (increase in size) and will potentially result in function and power closer to someone in their mid-20s. The older we get, the more we should expect to substitute hard endurance efforts for focussed, gym-based resistance training – it should become as natural as renewing our prescription for our reading glasses and very similarly predicated. There's also mounting evidence that maintaining muscle mass and function as we get older prevents central adiposity (fat stores) as well as reducing insulin resistance. Cycling physician Dr David Hulse, in a recent lecture that discussed sarcopenia, disclosed a little known fact about resistance training which helps individuals who are in rehab after trauma or injury: 'When you provide a stimulus in one limb, you switch on the anabolic genes in your whole body, to provide some adaptive training effect into areas that aren't being used.'

Hence, if you use weights on your left leg only, because your right leg is injured, there will be a strengthening response in the right leg as well. There is a popular picture on the internet showing a 70-year-old and a 40-year-old triathlete who have similar muscle bulk and fat deposits. By contrast, the picture also shows a 74-year-old sedentary man who has very little usable muscle mass and instead has an unhealthy burden of fat (adipose tissue layers). The 40-year-old and the 70-year-old may have similar cross-sectional muscle bulk, but it's safe to assume that the 40-year-old will be deriving much of the muscle mass from a rich density of muscle fibres, while the 70-year-old will have lost a substantial amount of fibres but has compensated very well by making the remaining ones bigger and stronger. So resistance training may not help with telomere length, and therefore ageing at a cellular level, but it has a hugely transformational effect on long-term strength, performance and function.

I remember racing a criterium when I was in my early 40s. As I rode around in the bunch waiting for the race to take shape, I was approached by an old teammate whom I had last seen 15 years before. Often bike races start quite gently, and you find yourself riding around at 40km/h having a coffee morning-style natter. Mick had raced competitively since he was a kid and was a wily rider and great sprinter if it came down to a bunch gallop. It was great to see him and chat, although ever the racer, I also made a note to myself to make sure he was not in the final selection at the end! Mick went on to lament his declining form: 'I'm nearly 60 now. I just don't have the explosive power anymore. It's my jump that has totally gone. I don't know what to do about it.'

And so it had. Natural-born sprinters in cycling are often quite lazy in my experience. They are born with a leg full of fast-twitch power and, as a consequence, often rely on one strategy to win a race. Namely, hope that the race stays together, goal hang at the end, find the right wheel in the last 400m and then unleash their race-winning blast. Mick had suffered from age-related sarcopenia in the last 15 years. And he had neither offset the worst effects by resistance training, nor had he switched training to boost his aerobic capacity to expand his racing repertoire with new strategies. When the race heated up, as it inevitably did, he could just about hide and hang on but could take no leading role. It came down to a bunch sprint, in which he inevitably didn't take part. I was just aware at the time that my own top-end was slightly blunted, and harder to access when I needed it. There are lessons that we can all learn from Mick's loss of muscle bulk and power, and it's a common theme with sprinters in the professional peloton also – they rarely adapt and find new strategies to win races once their explosive powder dampens.

We'll find out in more detail a little later in this chapter which hormonal mechanisms contribute to age-related sarcopenia.

The midlife skeleton

'Loaded bone is good bone.'

Stewart Tucker, spine surgeon

The cyclist's skeleton story is nuanced – the truth is that cyclists tend to struggle with their bones. Firstly, because we tend to fall off our bikes and break them, and secondly, because occasionally our skeletons lack the essential bone mineral density (BMD) of even extremely sedentary populations. Several studies have shown that cyclists tend to have lower BMD than age-matched controls, right across the age spectrums.

It's quite often the case after a cycling crash that we find an athlete has an underlying predisposition for their bones to fracture badly even under relatively superficial trauma. At Cyclefit, hip trauma and fractures are so common, with our amateur and professional clients, that we've developed a structured protocol to support a swift rehabilitation. Hip and pelvis injuries can be difficult for professional riders to fully recover from – witness Chris Froome's struggle to recapture full power after his crash in 2019, and Andy Schleck's debilitating pelvis injury sustained in the 2012 Critérium du Dauphiné. Furthermore, cyclists, especially professionals, often have low body and muscle mass, which would otherwise have a protective effect when a rider has an accident.

Many clients start off in an amended rehab position, and then when they are cleared by their medical team to return to riding, will move to a dedicated 'rehab bike' that they use out on the road. A rehab position will focus on preserving an open hip and as much space as possible at the top of the pedalstroke between the torso and the upper leg, utilising a shorter crank and higher handle-bar position. Top-level racers are often mortified by the specific adaptions that we make to help restore them to full function, but most also come to love their rehab bike and often keep it set up just in case.

The mineral referred to in 'BMD' is one of the best known, calcium. And our bones are overwhelmingly the biggest stores of calcium in our bodies. As well as being the building block for strong skeletal bones, calcium has a role in an impressive array of bodily functions – regulating heart rhythms, and impacting on blood clotting (calcium ions are integral in the activation of the blood thickening process post-injury), as well as nerve signalling and cellular function. Calcium is one of our body's most treasured and essential minerals and a deficit has implications outside of healthy bone mass.

There are two essential waypoints, in terms of bone health or lack of it – the first is called osteopenia and the second is called osteoporosis.

Osteoporosis is an imbalance between how much bone is being renewed and how much bone is being absorbed. Bone absorption is a transfer of minerals from the bone into the blood to facilitate vital body processes – this is a constant and natural process of regeneration. If osteogenesis (bone growth) is sufficiently low, our bone mass and density declines to the point our bones are at risk of fracture under stress. Calcium as a mineral is so valuable for our general health and well-being that if there's not enough of it in our blood, the body will simply absorb it out of our bones to compensate. The body is making the decision that general body health and function ultimately trumps bone density and strength.

Osteopenia is a midway point between a healthy BMD and being osteoporotic, where the bones are clinically weakened. Osteopenia is an important marker for doctors because it demonstrates that someone is metabolising more calcium from bones than can be replaced – in simple terms the body is using more bone than it's making. This isn't a healthy equilibrium because BMD naturally declines as we age, so the overall trend would be a slide towards osteoporosis and substantial skeletal weakening.

We reach peak BMD at around the age of 30, depending upon diet and lifestyle choices. At that age, men have about 1500g of skeletal calcium, while women have about 1250g. The decline in men's calcium levels is fairly constant, but for women, the decline steepens as they go through menopause at around age 50, then levels off again as they head into their 60s.

It sounds obvious, but all of our calcium comes from our food – if we don't eat enough calcium-rich foods the body will automatically scavenge bone stores to bring the body back into homeostasis (physiological balance). The absorption of calcium in our bodies is indelibly associated with an increasingly prescient compound called vitamin D. Low Vitamin D levels, at the time of writing, are thought to be linked to the risk of developing adverse Covid-19 symptoms – several studies are hurrying to establish this link. Vitamin D is actually not a vitamin at all, it's a steroid-derived hormone that we either synthesise in the skin or ingest as food – typically fatty fish, eggs or milk. Unlike vitamins C or B, which we cannot easily store in our bodies and so need to regularly replenish, vitamin D is stored in our fat, meaning we can build up a supply in the summer that will last us through the winter. Naturally, this is easier in hot and sunny countries than it is in colder climes, where it's easier to become vitamin D-deprived, which in turn will compromise the absorption of calcium. Many athletes living in less sunny climates now take vitamin D during the winter months. It's worth saying that athletes who are most at risk of lower BMD are the ones whose low weight gives a performance advantage and whose dietary intake may be tightly controlled. Poor BMD has been linked to individuals who are in energy deficit – they are routinely expending more energy than they are consuming. Not your typical midlife cyclist (well, not this one anyway.)

One of the main factors contributing to low BMD in cyclists is an almost total lack of impact, or sheer mechanical loading, through their bodies. The very thing that protects our ageing knees, backs and hips may also expose us to a risk of poor bone strength, as cycling physician Dave Hulse, a pro-team doctor, explains: 'Bones respond positively to loads and stress by increasing their mineral content by pulling in calcium content from the diet and bloodstream, provided of course that there's enough available.'

This reminds me of my own experience a couple of years ago when I had to undergo spine fusion surgery from T12 to L2 (thoracic vertebrae number 12 and lumbar vertebrae number 2 – often referred to as the thoracic-lumbar junction). The operation involved putting in a titanium spacer from the front via my ribcage, and titanium rods on the rear of my spine. Twelve or so hours afterwards, the surgeon, Stewart Tucker, 'invited' me to stand and walk a few steps. When he saw the look on my face, he quietly encouraged me by saying, 'loaded bone is good bone'. He knew that even so soon after the procedure the bone was ready to start healing and growing again to complete the fusion process. I dutifully stood up and tottered around the ward. I then proceeded to walk a million steps over the next couple of months to provide the best bone-growth stimulus possible. Even had I been able to ride a bike, cycling would have done very little to promote osteogenic stimulus or the required bone growth and long-term healing.

It sounds counter-intuitive but should all midlife cyclists be thinking about dropping a couple of training sessions in favour of running or fast walking, and weight training? Running and weight training will exert the appropriate loading and mechanical stress that will, in turn, encourage increased mineral density in our bones. Remember that running will also work on general aerobic/anaerobic conditioning and was positively implicated in encouraging telomere length, while resistance training will also clearly offset the age-related effects of sarcopenia. The road to becoming a great cyclist in middle age and beyond may well involve doing less cycling in favour of other activities.

But in my experience of working with thousands of midlife cyclists at Cyclefit, many of them are migrating from sports such as running, squash and rugby, because they are injured, and future participation in those activities is painful or not advised. So, what should we do if we cannot run anymore? Graham Anderson, my old friend and colleague, is one of the UK's most experienced elite sports physiotherapists. Graham has a wonderfully rational stance on what cyclists should do to support their sport. For him it comes down to one simple thing – cyclists don't have enough 'dynamic chaos' in their 'activity diet'. We're very comfortable with low-impact, micro-controlled, repetitive movement, like pedalling in predictable circles, held up by two wheels and a bicycle frame. But make us stand literally and metaphorically on our own two feet or, even worse, on one foot, and our wheels fall off. For Graham, making cyclists stronger and more resilient is all about adding 'chaos' into our exercise routines. And this can be a simple thing to do – I became one of Graham's clients when I was in rehab after my back surgery and well on my way to recovery. But it was clear I shouldn't run anymore, even though recovery was going well and I needed to push forwards to increase fitness and function. Graham advised me to deliberately walk off the forest track and onto rougher ground, so each step was, by definition a different length and therefore not predictable. Chaotic. I progressed to deliberately negotiating routes that involved traversing logs and streams and hills – the energy requirement and loading was hugely increased with Graham's chaotic prescription, but I felt the benefit in terms of healing, strength and function. If you cannot run or have been advised that you shouldn't, I recommend the Anderson Protocol along with a guided weights programme.

There are other factors that are thought to negatively and progressively affect our bone mineral density. One that has recently come to the fore is calcium mineral loss through sweating and dehydration. Studies have found that enough calcium is lost through sweating to cause a potential problem, when combined with other factors such as reduced dietary intake, age-related decline and low-impact exercise burden. Does that ring any bells for anyone? Are you a post-50 athlete, who trains extensively, or even exclusively, indoors in a sweaty environment? Are you also on a long-term negative weight management programme and, if female, going through the menopause? If you scored more than two out of that list of four, it may be advisable to supplement with vitamin D and calcium or, better still, have a DEXA scan (low-dose x-ray bone densitometry scan) and a vitamin D blood test.

For the midlife cyclist, the steps to take to maintain good bone health, in the face of normal age-related loss, are relatively simple: a balanced diet, a possible vitamin D supplement if you're sunshine-deprived or a vegan and don't eat dairy, avoiding protracted cycling indoors in hot sweaty spaces, and starting resistance training and/or running once or twice a week to create the mechanical stress that will provide osteogenic stimulus in order to create more bone mineral density.

Midlife joints, tendons and ligaments

Other than fractures when we fall off our bikes or turbo-trainers, or creeping osteopenia that lies dormant until it's discovered and treated, not much goes wrong inside the bones themselves. As Alex Fugallo, ex-international 400m runner and forensic osteopath, points out, most of the problems that become more prevalent as athletes age and try to maintain or even increase their activity levels, relate to joints, tendons and ligaments. The irony of being an osteopath who spends all day treating midlifers' joints, tendons and ligaments, and not bones, isn't lost on him.

Tendons and ligaments are strong, fibrous connective structures that assist with joint movement and stabilisation. Tendons join muscles to bones and are therefore involved in the transfer of power and energy. For example, our biggest and strongest tendon is the Achilles, which connects the calf muscles to the heel bone (calcaneus). When the calf muscles contract, the Achilles tendon 'plantar flexes' the foot (pulls the heel up) and enables us to stand up on our toes. The Achilles tendon has to have incredible tensile strength (it can pull up to 900kg) because it's controlling our entire body weight. Ligaments are similar to tendons in that they are also formed of collagen-based fibrous connective tissue, but they only join bone to bone (not muscle to bone). Probably the best-known and most troublesome ligament is the anterior cruciate ligament (ACL). The ACL and larger posterior cruciate ligament (PCL) attach the thigh bone (femur) to your shin bone (tibia). The role of both the ACL and PCL is to stabilise the knee joint under load. The ACL is smaller than the PCL, and has an inferior blood supply. But the ACL's Achilles heel, if you'll forgive the clumsy metaphor, is that it's vulnerable to side trauma and twisting, such as being tackled from the side in rugby, or a skiing accident. Folk like Graham and Alex spend their long winter months working with clients who have injured or even snapped their ACL or PCL. As a point of reference, we have many clients who race bikes at the highest level without an intact ACL, and I have never heard of anyone snapping their

ACL or PCL as a result of riding or falling from a bike – but I probably will now.

Nature, or evolution, is pretty clever – or should I say ruthlessly efficient? It has found a way to arrange the collagen fibres that make up both tendons and ligaments to resist or transfer forces, in much the same way that carbon fibre is arranged in a bike frame to transfer power or add flex and comfort. In fact, the carbon metaphor is a pretty sound one – carbon fibre is a matrix, or composite, of aramid strands that are highly organised and kept in place by being impregnated in resin. To be clear, all the tensile or structural strength in carbon fibre comes from the fibre part of the matrix and not the resin part. Tendons and ligaments are also a composite of highly organised and very specific collagen fibres in different ratios according to the loading patterns they have to resist or transmit. For example, the Achilles tendon changes its role when we walk or run – as we drive our heel down at the beginning of a step the Achilles stretches, and as we toe-off at the end of a step, the Achilles acts a little like a spring as it releases energy. Kangaroos have adapted this principle to an even greater degree, by evolving phenomenal tendons that act like giant leaf springs, allowing them to cruise at 50km/h with 8m leaps.

But what happens to human ligament and tendon structures as we get older? Believe it or not, this isn't yet fully understood. But we do know that the composition of the collagen fibre matrix can become a little more disorganised (especially post-injury), like some of the carbon fibres in your bicycle frame suddenly pointing the wrong way and resisting the wrong forces, resulting in the bottom bracket swinging around as you apply power, or the seat stays becoming stiff over bumps. Blood supply (vascular) changes have also been recorded in ligaments and tendons as we progressively age, which has implications for healing and biomechanical function. There's also a reduction in the vital 'mechanotransduction' function, whereby mechanical stress inputs are converted into electrochemical activity. So back to Alex Fugallo, who has observed that the operating window of stress and recovery response is much smaller as we get older. This means that if the load is too small, you don't get the restorative effect that you need; too large, and the structures risk breaking down again. Alex also tries to manage athlete expectation early in the treatment pathway – muscles, ligaments and bones normally achieve primary healing within six weeks, but tendons can take up to six months. Tendon recovery – patella, Achilles and rotator cuff, for example – is a particularly fast-moving subject. But what can we do to help as midlife athletes?

Firstly – and of primary importance – we can make sure that we don't allow our muscles to atrophy because that creates abnormal loading on the tendons and ligaments. So, it's vital that we actively resist sarcopenia with specific resistance training. Remember, we'll lose muscle fibres as we grow older, so the only way to preserve muscle bulk and therefore strength is to make the remaining fibres more trained and functional.

Secondly, we must make sure we're correctly calibrated for every activity we're involved with. In cycling, patella and Achilles tendonitis are almost entirely due to incorrect bike set-up, resulting in adverse loading on the structures involved (see chapter 5). Similarly, Achilles issues in running are almost always the consequence of poor conditioning, technique and/or incorrect foot posture and support.

Midlife hormones

In athletic terms, 50 is the new 30. There are plenty of us out there trying to extract more performance from our bodies in our mid-50s and 60s than at any other time in our lives. As a consequence, we need to be mindful of the forces we are opposing as we try to roll the performance rock back up the steep hill. And one of the strongest gravitational pulls is provided by our endocrine systems, and the hormones that are under its control. And if that sentence just made you unexpectedly emotional and tearful, feel free to blame your hormones.

If we want to maximise our performance into middle age and well beyond, we could all do a lot worse than marry an endocrinologist – for these clinicians truly hold the keys to the performance castle. The endocrine system is a network of glands that play an essential role in keeping the entire body in homeostasis (physiological equilibrium). Hormones are the endocrine system's biological text messages, sent out to the furthest reaches of our bodies and organs. Whereas the nervous system uses electrical signals, the endocrine system uses chemical messages to signal that a biochemical recalibration is required somewhere else in the body. For example, the adrenal glands are situated at the top of your kidneys and produce the well-known hormone adrenaline, which signals that heart rate and blood pressure should rise in response to a potentially stressful or dangerous situation. The signal is sent out by the adrenal gland, but the messages are received and acted upon in various parts of the body – increased output at the heart, dilation of the pupils in our eyes and even increased blood sugar levels, for example.

The general trend is that most hormone levels decline as we age or, even if the quantity of the signalling hormone doesn't change, then sometimes the receptor is less sensitive or the organ responsible for making the change is just less capable. The hormone, remember, is just a signalling agent for change to be acted upon by another part of the body. Sports endocrinologist Dr Nicky Keay says: 'Hormones start declining with age, in particular those that are important for gaining adaptive benefits from training – growth hormone and testosterone. These are gradual declines but for women there's an abrupt stop of female hormones at menopause, which often has a big impact on cycling performance.'

Let's evaluate the key hormonal changes that have the biggest impact on high-level training and competition as we get older. This is a slightly naïve proposition because our body's performance is predicated on complex and interlinked functioning between all of our key systems. So, for example, we won't be talking much (if at all) about aldosterone, which is a steroid hormone secreted by the adrenal gland and has a vital homeostatic role in the maintenance of salt balance and hydration. While we can all see how vital healthy aldosterone levels might be when we're halfway up Alpe d'Huez in 35-degree heat, its link to performance is secondary and peripheral.

The 'big three' hormonal shifts that affect performance and our general health, well-being and sense of ourselves are: testosterone, oestrogen and growth hormone. But we'll also look at our changing relationship with insulin as we progressively age. And we may mention a little-known hormone called melatonin.

Testosterone

Testosterone is one of the best-known hormones and is actually found in both men and women, but is the primary male sex hormone and consequently has a huge impact on both health and performance. Testosterone gradually declines as we age, in both men and women (especially post-menopause). In men, levels decline at around one per cent per year after the age of 30, and as a consequence men can expect to have around half the testosterone in their 70s and 80s as they did in their 20s. Does that matter, and is there anything we can do about it? The easy answers are: yes and err, somewhat. Testosterone has a key metabolic role in many of our body's functions. A lack of testosterone can lead to:

- Sarcopenia – age-related muscle-loss
- Osteopenia and osteoporosis – loss of bone
- Increased lipid stores – testosterone helps us keep fat stores controlled
- Decrease in cognitive function – loss of alertness and sharpness
- Low libido – declining sex drive, not normally an issue on a bike.

Declining testosterone levels is a controversial subject at the moment, and not just for male midlife athletes looking to preserve a good balance between training and health. Under discussion among scientists are:

- What constitutes abnormally low or high readings?
- Is it OK to use testosterone replacement therapy (TRT) to boost levels back to normal?
- Should we all be taking TRT as we get older to maintain the levels that we enjoyed when we were younger?

It will come as no surprise that TRT potentially comes at a massive physical cost for some of us midlife athletes. (Back to the background context of our genetic irrelevance again – the chances of us even being alive post 50 in the ancestral environment were millions to one.) Testosterone levels decline past 30 probably because in evolutionary terms there has never been a selective pressure to preserve them. By age 30 in every other era, we would already have bred (or not) and almost certainly died already. But just because we can supplement our testosterone level back to that found in our 19-year-old selves doesn't mean that we should. Call me a killjoy if you must, but I'm just not sure it's advisable, or even desirable, for us to wander the planet with the hormone levels of a teenager when we are in our 50s. The risks of TRT prescription in middle-aged men are thought to run a whole spectrum that includes: increased risk of cardiovascular disease, prostate cancer and even a biological dependence (i.e. inhibited production of natural testosterone). We'll come back to what steps we can naturally put in place to mitigate declining testosterone levels at the end of this chapter.

Oestrogen

Oestrogen is the primary female sex hormone. Although it's found in both men and women, it's much more prevalent and powerful for female physiology and psychology. Unlike in men, however, whose rate of hormone decline is at least linear, in women, the rate of decline of oestrogen (and progesterone) is much faster during menopause, before slowing post-menopause. The ramifications of declining female sex hormones for women is more complex and nuanced than testosterone loss is for men. Dr Keay again: 'We are living longer, together with an increase in age-group participation. For a woman, up to third of her life will be spent in a menopausal state.'

Shifts in oestrogen can affect health and performance in the following ways:

- Bone mineral density tends to drop with hormonal declines.
- Oestrogen is intrinsically anti-inflammatory and has a positive effect on the female immune system. Some of this effect will be lost.
- There's potential for muscle loss and loss of strength during and post-menopause.
- Oestrogen is thought to have a protective effect on the heart, especially during high-level endurance training and competition (see chapter 3). Some of this effect may be lost.
- Up to two-thirds of women report sleep interruption, or loss of quality rest.
- There is evidence that hormonal changes before and during menopause can result in more visceral or belly fat as women move away from their reproductive years and oestrogen and progesterone levels decline.

All of this can look a little depressing when expressed as a downward slanting shopping list, but exercise, and especially high doses of the right exercise, can have a miraculous ameliorating effect for both men and women.

Hormone replacement therapy (HRT) for women is much less controversial than TRT is for men; and as a consequence, many women choose this treatment pathway. The benefit to risk proposition of HR7 to TR7 seems to make the former more compelling than the latter. The obvious exceptions would be where an individual is clinically deficient in testosterone – i.e. androgen deficiency of the ageing male (ADAM) – and corrective therapy is medically indicated, directed and supervised.

Growth hormone

Now back to my flippant comment earlier about why those serious about performance at any cost should marry an endocrinologist. With testosterone and growth hormone (plus erythropoietin, or EPO) you have *The Complete Cheat's Perfect Cookbook!* Hormones are the first stone that drug cheats look under, once they move away from the blunt impact of amphetamine usage. And the most abused would be a naturally occurring agent called human growth hormone (HGH, or simply GH). HGH is a naturally occurring hormone that's secreted in the pituitary gland, which is at the base of the brain. HGH reaches its peak when we go through puberty and inevitably decreases at around 1–2 per cent per annum after 30 years of age, for the rest of our lives. Growth hormone signals receptor cells all around our body to reproduce and grow, so it's no surprise that HGH as a supplement is the number one target on the hit list of the World Anti-Doping Agency (WADA). Our natural HGH production fundamentally makes us bigger, stronger and physically more capable. Just scan the physiological properties of declining natural HGH levels:

- An increase in body lipids (fats) – especially visceral (trunk) fats
- A decrease in lean muscle bulk
- A reduction in aerobic capacity
- A decrease in bone mineral formation
- A decrease in EPO production in the kidneys
- A neural decline, possibly affecting cognition and alertness
- A possible deterioration of the immune system

When you see that list, it makes you wonder why we're all not taking HGH like statins, vitamin D and HRT – what would we all not want boosted in that physiological shopping list? Stronger, fitter, sharper, more resilient – and libido didn't even make it into HGH's greatest hits. It's abundantly clear why HGH was the booster of choice for professional cyclists in the 1990s and early 2000s. So, if HGH is a potential fountain of youth, it seems cruel to deny us its miraculous benefits. But early studies have shown that there are possible side effects from HGH supplementation – joint pain, fluid retention and increased cancer risk, especially prostate cancer. In the same way that it's perfectly possible to take my first ever car, a 1966 Triumph Herald 1250, and pop in a turbocharger to instantly double its horsepower from 51bhp to over 100bhp, common sense tells me that even if the engine survived (it broke down constantly with a mere 51bhp) the brakes, steering and suspension would be quickly and dangerously overwhelmed. So just because we can, doesn't always mean we should. And anyway, there are proven, healthy and successful ways for us to tune our engines without resorting to dramatic high-risk strategies. Just not necessarily for Triumph Heralds.

Buy three, get two free

I briefly want to mention two other hormones – insulin and melatonin, which are linked to our metabolism. Insulin, and its binary twin glucagon, are opposing signalling hormones, and both are secreted by the pancreas. The former decreases blood glucose levels and the latter increases them. This is a perfect example of contrary chemical signalling being used to hold the body in perfect homeostasis. Doctors have found that fasted glucose levels tend to rise over the age of 50, possibly because the body gets less efficient at metabolising glucose into the muscle cells, liver and fat stores. A fasted state is one where you have run out of food that is waiting to be digested and therefore release as energy. It's therefore possible that the hormone signal is being transmitted but is being poorly implemented within the intestine by the receptor cells. However, it's perfectly possible also that the amount of insulin being produced may also be in decline. Unlike testosterone and oestrogen, however, which have most certainly evolved to reduce as we age, this isn't the case with insulin, but we can say that our sensitivity to sugar and how it's metabolised becomes more complicated as we age.

Melatonin is a weird little hormone secreted by the pineal gland in our brains. The pineal gland is large in children and then atrophies incrementally post-puberty. This makes total sense if you think about how younger children's psychology dramatically changes when they are exhausted and just need to sleep – all too often their last words of the day are, 'but I'm not tired!' before surrendering to the deepest slumber! Not everything is known about the pineal gland or the mysterious little hormone that it releases. But there's a consensus that it takes a role in regulating our circadian rhythms and sleep architecture and that this becomes more compromised as we get older.

The ageing hormones toolkit

Is there any way back from that woe-filled scroll of vital hormonal loss and the associated incremental decline in our vitality, performance and general health? Before you bulk order testosterone patches, HRT and shots of HGH, there's a very practical and well-proven package of measures that we can and should all implement to ameliorate age-related hormonal shifts.

Reversing or mitigating the effects of hormonal decline as a veteran athlete can generally be placed under the neutral flag of 'deciding to live well'. Put another way, we can either fall into a negative performance cascade where the dominoes of poor diet, low exercise and bad sleep patterns fall over to create a surge of poor health and low physical competence. Or we can create a positive cascade, where we work with our bodies to constructively fortify against the worst that nature and evolution is throwing at us. In effect, we can't stop the cellular fuse from burning, but we can lengthen it and slow it down. Dr Keay spells it out: 'The main stimuli for GH release are exercise and sleep . . . focus on strength work off bike to support both GH and testosterone production. Resistance work supports favourable body composition.' Here's the low-down:

- **Start resistance training**. Strength training and intense intervals will increase the levels of both HGH and testosterone and also offset the negative dynamic of weight gain and muscle loss. Cyclists who stick to pure endurance training could be contributing to a decline in testosterone, in particular. Midlife athletes should drop one or two bike sessions for structured resistance training. The benefits are real, proven and unambiguous – increased muscle mass, as well as higher bone mineral, testosterone and HGH levels.
- **Get better sleep**. Drs Hulse and Keay both flag up sleep as the health wonder panacea. Managing a good sleep balance increases the production of HGH and testosterone, as well as managing stress and increasing recovery post-training. Remember Team Sky spending fortunes on their Tour de France sleep trailer/pod for whoever was their designated team leader? Team Sky were also one of the first teams to transport their own pillows and mattresses around for every rider – they were the first to understand that sleep was substantially more than a 'marginal gain'. The aphorism 'sleep like a baby' has physiological resonance because babies are hardwired to sleep better than midlifers because of their comparatively high melatonin levels. But us midlife athletes also need superb sleep architecture to recover and maintain hormonal health. This will almost certainly involve conscious changes to diet and

lifestyle, such as avoiding alcohol (known to disrupt REM) and sugar (especially at the end of the day), and practising mindfulness to reduce stress.

- **Reduce sugar intake**. HGH levels are quite glucose sensitive. Reducing sugar intake will offset insulin sensitivity changes as well as help HGH production levels. Since HGH is substantially produced at night time, try to avoid sugary snacks before you go to bed. Reducing sugars will also control fat levels, which themselves can also inhibit testosterone and HGH levels. We'll go into much more detail in chapter seven.

- **Monitor vitamin D levels**. Low levels of the hormone are thought to be associated with inhibited testosterone production.

- **Don't compromise on recovery – ever!** We ought to modify our training regime as we get older to receive the best adaptive response and maximise hormonal balance. Dr Keay says: 'An important factor is adequate recovery between training sessions.' Sedentary people aren't active enough – midlife athletes tend to be too active or not active in the right way. We need more and better structured recovery time as we get older. Doing the same as we always have will embed fatigue and negative metabolic and hormonal dynamics.

- **Reduce general stress**. Stress induces the release of a hormone called cortisol, which inhibits the production of testosterone. To build muscle and performance you need to calm down.

Heart and lung midlife changes

One of this book's calling cards is a detailed and uncompromising review of age-related decline and change in the male and female veteran heart, to establish the risks associated with high intensity and high duration cycling. As a consequence, I'll confine myself here to a scant overview of what's happening to our engine rooms as we age but still want to maintain active participation in high-level cycling and competition. Much of this you'll already know from your own experience, or sense from the general thread of the earlier dialogue around bones, muscles, tendons and hormones. Lifelong exercisers and data-trackers will have a different view of their experience to folk who have only started their athletic career recently. If you are a lifelong athlete, you will have performance markers that you will have almost certainly monitored over years or decades, such as your favourite climb. Mine is called Holloway Lane and connects Turville to Northend, in the Chilterns. Everything about the way I negotiate the two miles and 500 feet of vertical ascent has changed from my racing days. Previously I would attack the foot of the climb and then attempt to hang onto the pace up the steeper sections, out of the saddle, trying to always change up through the gears. Now my primary endeavour is to hold a constant effort, moving repeatedly between standing and seated. Of course I am also significantly slower than my racing days, but my motivation and methodology have also changed. But interestingly I love that little tunnel of trees and high-sided banks more than I ever have.

An interesting question, of course, would be, when did the performance deflection begin? I remember very well following the same training pattern year-on-year and still being able to compete in shorter elite races and, on a good day, with a fair wind, could come away with a good result. At the age of 41, I rode a 100km race at Goodwood on a blisteringly hot day, and came second to an elite rider who had chipped off the front. I came second because I didn't see him go off the breakaway group I was in (I still have no idea how I missed it) and not because I lacked aerobic fitness. The next year, at the age of 42, I started to find things more difficult – I needed to train more just to tread water and maintain my racing weight. I know now that this was the ante-room of age-related VO_2 Max decline. (This was a lab ramp test of how much volume (V) of oxygen (O2) your body could use as a proportion of your bodyweight in kilogrames in one minute.) I was never again capable of contesting a race at that level. VO_2 Max is the holy grail of endurance sport, and always has been. VO_2 measures how efficient your heart and lungs are at converting oxygen into energy that can be used by your muscles. It's quite literally a measurement of how much oxygen your body can utilise in millilitres, per kilogram of body weight per minute – giving us the magic equation, mL/kg/min. Functional threshold power (FTP) has recently stolen the halo of VO_2, but FTP is a trifling downstream function of VO_2. The ability of the body to utilise oxygen efficiently was one of the biological facets that helped us persistence hunt in the ancestral environment in the sense that we traded outright speed for endurance when we evolved from four legs to two legs. And it's now this combination of bipedal efficiency and ability to function aerobically over time and distance that we use to scale the Col du Galibier on a bicycle.

In aged matched longitudinal studies, sedentary folk were compared to top endurance athletes over an eight-year period. The VO_2 Max of the sedentary group declined by a significant 12 per cent, from an average of 33.9 to 30.6 mL/kg/min. The athlete group only declined by around 5.5 per cent, from an average of 54.0 to 51.8 mL/kg/min. Many aspects of this kind of research – which all seem to show the same trends – are fascinating. Firstly, the athletes' VO_2 numbers are 70 per cent higher than the sedentary group – the athletes are almost a different species. Secondly, the rate of decline in the athletes' VO_2 is less than half that of the sedentary folk. Not only do athletes enjoy better health and function overall but by exercising they are mitigating over half of their decline. That's little short of astounding.

Diesels and hummingbirds

But why does VO_2 decline at all with age? Why do I struggle to attack the climb from Turville to Northend with quite the same gusto that I did only 20 years ago? It all comes down to declining maximum heart rates. We've all heard the finger-in-the-air '220 minus your age' as a broad litmus of your theoretical maximum heart rate. This crude algorithm may miss the fact that some of us are low-revving diesels and always will be, and some of us are high-revving hummingbirds – but the rate of decline is real and uniform. The lowering of the maximum heart rate gives the athlete a smaller operating cardiovascular window in which to operate. If we take your car engine and put a limiter on its maximum number of revs – for example, 6000rpm down to 4500rpm – the power drop will be marked and irrevocable. It's exactly the same with the heart – there's simply less oxygenated blood being pumped to the muscles from the left ventricle side of the heart. And just so you know, the solution isn't to pop on a turbocharger – see my earlier analogy about my 1966 Triumph Herald 1250.

Strategies for maintaining your VO_2 Max

Here are the basic rules for keeping that VO_2 Max as high as possible for as long as possible:

- **Don't get fat.** VO_2, by definition, is a function of your weight. Excess fat contributes nothing to performance and acts as an active and dynamic drag on VO_2 – recent studies have shown that preserving lean muscle bulk as we get older is vital to maintaining a high VO_2.
- **Keep training levels high.** But switch to multi-discipline activities, such as cross-training and resistance training. Don't do the very same thing you've always done and expect the same result year-on-year – you cannot fight evolution and your genes.
- **Keep going.** As we've seen, athletes halve their VO_2 decline against age-matched sedentary groups from 12 per cent to 5.5 per cent. Remember, it's been known for athletes to increase their VO_2 Max as they age, but they have to modify and

improve their training to offset declining heart rate potential. If you keep exercising in a rational way, you'll have a VO_2 that's significantly higher at age 55 than a sedentary 25 year old. We're the first generation in the history of mankind to enjoy that kind of midlife performance! This isn't at all trivial and is to be celebrated.

Perceptions, reactions and recall

We've established that our hardware is prone to some attritional deterioration if we don't deliberately offset the worst effects with structured lifestyle changes, such as training, sleep and diet. But does the software (our systems that are linked to perception and control, rather than physical power output and movement) also start to glitch as we age? Throughout my life I have enjoyed 20/20 vision but I'm now in a midlife sweet spot of being both short- and long-sighted all at the same time. I spend my whole life wearing one pair of glasses, with another pair pre-emptively poised on top of my head. Theoretically, therefore, there must be a precise focal length where I can see absolutely perfectly (I am yet to find it), as I transition from long to short and back again. I'm a textbook case – during the research for this book I would repeatedly discover some element of our physicality that hypothetically changes past 40, and almost without fail I could relate to it. As a result, I'm steeped in empathy. And so it is with our eyes – we tend to become long-sighted as we age, as the lens within the eye becomes harder and less flexible, and the muscles that control it become less effective. As a result, we perceive an increasingly blurry image, as we struggle to focus upon objects nearby or at a distance. I now ride with glasses, which can be a problem when it rains, or in early morning fog. I don't know of any training you can do to correct your eyes, so we're all limited to the options of:

- Prescription glasses and prescription cycling sunglasses – very important

- Laser surgery – I'm saving up
- Contact lenses – most pro cyclists go down this road and I'm not sure why I haven't, other than I'm not professional

Controlling a fast-moving bicycle over any terrain is a complex synaptic juggling exercise that uses a huge amount of cognitive ability – I'm personally convinced that this is one of the reasons why cycling is so good for us, and why indoor cycling, though sometimes sensible, isn't as mentally refreshing as outdoor cycling. However, when we ride at pace, our dominant sense is sight – we're only 2.5cm (1in) of quality rubber away from A&E at any one time, and we're making 95 per cent of our decisions by line of sight. My two top tips here are: get your eyes tested regularly; and make sure you have cycling-specific prescription sunglasses, if you need them. Our eyes will continue to decline as we age, and it happens largely below our conscious radar.

In a previous life, before I started to race and work with bicycles, I worked in the music industry. I spent many years either holed up in a studio or out on the road with artists at gigs every evening. As a consequence, I have exaggerated age-related hearing loss, as well as permanent tinnitus and a huge gap where my high-end frequency response should be. If we ever meet out on the road, be sure to shout in a deep voice if you want me to hear. Or just maybe I'll have got a hearing aid by then.

While our ear lobes unhelpfully get bigger as we gently age, our hearing, and specifically our high-end frequency response, fades incrementally. The cause is thought to be that the tiny hairs inside your inner ears, which turn sound waves into neural signals, die over time, and by way of a considerable genetic oversight aren't replaced. Hearing loss is therefore progressive and mostly inescapable. Strangely, as my hearing gets worse my tinnitus gets louder. A friend of mine – who also experiences tinnitus – and is dual-skilled as a psychotherapist and evolutionary psychologist – gave me the very best advice on this: 'Never give tinnitus any headspace to grow, don't think about it, or acknowledge it. We should never speak of it again.'

I'm not sure this is applicable to cycling in any way, but it's certainly a component of midlife ageing. I shall never speak of this aspect of ageing again, and nor should you.

Putting the cogs into cognition

I was wholly convinced, even before we started the research for this book, that cycling outside, on tarmac or off-road, is superb for mental health, cognition and short- and long-term memory. I've used cycling for decades as a mental church for regathering and recentering my thoughts and soul. It's one of the (many) reasons I dislike indoor cycling, because I think so many of the uplifting effects on mood and soul are conspicuously lacking.

As I mentioned in the previous section, riding a bike at pace, and especially in a group, is a mental and physical ballet of high-power outputs and fine machine control, mixed with intricate spatial and social awareness. For me, hard riding is as much of a cognitive high as it is a physical one. I remember chasing Jules, my Cyclefit colleague, down the backside of the Col du Glandon at 9/10th pace a few years ago. We have a similar descending style – fast, smooth and continually mixing up classic cornering with counter-steering techniques, so we were hitting the apexes inches apart from each other. It probably looked dangerous to anyone looking on, but we've raced with other for decades and know each other's style and strengths. Descending at 80km/h or more, we worked as hard mentally, descending, as we did climbing, physically. On a bike, the fine control comes through weighting through the pedals, and the orientation of your centre of gravity with the centrifugal forces of the wheels. It's the sheer amount of data that's being processed at such pace that gives such an endorphin rush, I'm sure.

But does the research and science back me up? Well, in fact it does – numerous studies have repeatedly shown that cardiovascular exercise prevents cognitive decline and may also reverse some of the worst aspects of neural ageing by supporting something called 'synaptic plasticity', which improves the quality of neurons in our brains and how they communicate with each other. Which is precisely how it feels to me when I ride down an alpine pass.

Synaptic plasticity in neuroscience is the process of storing and retrieving vital information in the brain as a consequence of the individual neurons dynamically communicating with each other. Synaptic plasticity is something we should seek to preserve and enjoy as we mature. The research seems to indicate that exercise increases blood flow and levels of neurotransmitters such as serotonin, which helps the brain work more efficiently, as well as having a protective effect on neural networks.

Other studies have shown that high-level exercise actively helps brain volume and 'grey matter' reduction. One study conducted by researchers at Wake Forest University in North Carolina used 'peak' exercise on 65 previously sedentary men and women. At the end of the six-month trial, the researchers found significantly less tau proteins in their blood and spinal fluid. Tau is a component of amyloid plaques, which are thought to contribute to Alzheimer's disease. All of the test subjects also scored significantly higher in cognitive tests. The research authors went out of their way to point out that the exercise had to be as vigorous as the test subjects could reasonably tolerate. I'm pretty sure a climb and descent of the Col du Glandon would have achieved much the same results.

The study came to an unusually definitive conclusion: 'The results indicate that aerobic exercise is more effective than any currently approved medication in forestalling Alzheimer's disease.'

Most of us ride bicycles fast because we intrinsically love the activity – we appreciate the very nature of the thing itself in that moment. Riding along forest tracks in autumn on damp leaves, miles away from home while testing yourself against both terrain and topography – very few things in life can be as good for you physically and emotionally. Some people cycle for the perceived fitness and health improvements that they get – any spiritual effect or excitement is a welcome secondary benefit. Not many of us, I wager, cycle to offset the effects of age-related physical and cognitive decline. But these miraculous effects are accepted now. We can't stop the years clicking by, but we can slow the genetic clock, by simply doing what we love in a slightly more structured and reasoned manner.

2

IT IS ABOUT THE BIKE

The fact that the basic design and dynamics of bicycles and cycling were devised by obviously inebriated Victorians around the time of HG Wells and Thomas Hardy shouldn't put us off – it's a very fine thing if we understand its wonderful qualities but also its limitations. You may well ask why the design has endured, largely unchanged, for 140 years, if it is fundamentally flawed? Or put another way, if the bicycle hadn't previously existed, would we design the same machine in 2020? The modern bicycle persists, largely unchanged in terms of riding dynamics and biomechanics, for two essential reasons. Firstly, because it's good enough – it takes professional riders 3000km around France every July at average speeds of over 40km/h at one end of the spectrum, and millions of commuters and utility riders quickly and quietly about their business, at the other. Secondly, the Union Cycliste Internationale (UCI) enshrined the modern bicycle into its current form by banning Charles Mochet's world-beating design in 1933 (allegedly under pressure from the car and bicycle industries). This was effectively a 'speciation event' – the bicycle went from a potentially improvable instrument into a cultural object that now had to conform to arbitrarily applied rules. It had become a species.

This speciation event took place when designer Charles Mochet and local racer Francis Faure decided to take on Oscar Egg's 1914 Hour Record of 44.247km. Egg's record had stood for 20 years and was universally considered to be unbeatable. Faure was the equivalent of a second category racer and was not given much chance of taking the record at an open event against a few professional riders, who were also making attempts. Mochet and Faure were careful to get the blessing of the all-powerful UCI for his Velocar 'recumbant' design. On the day, Faure was mocked by his fellow competitors. But Mochet had done his homework and the hilarity stopped once Faure's track speed was clear. By the end of the hour, Faure and Mochet had added almost a whole kilometre to Egg's unassailable record, at 45.028km.

Charles Mochet's ultimate dream was to provide low-cost, sustainable transport to France as the country struggled with a lack of resources, particularly petrol, following the First World War. The Faure Velocar gave him proof of concept to launch microcars powered by pedal, or a mixture of pedal and motor assist. The dashing of his dream is our speciation event. The UCI, under lobby from the French bicycle manufacturers and the car industry, immediately annulled Faure and Mochet's record. At the same time, they also banned the design from all competition. Two months later, the UCI prescriptively laid down very precise criteria for the definition of a bike.

The ease with which Faure took Oscar Egg's hour record terrified the French car and bicycle industries. They used the blunt power of the UCI to define what a bicycle was and still is. This eradicated the record and destroyed Mochet's plans. He died a year later.

This UCI definition was essentially the same criteria that the Wright brothers used in 1895. A lazy bicycle industry now had little need to move from this arbitrary set of random criteria because it had been set in stone by the UCI. The species of the bicycle was from that point forward effectively enshrined. The UCI has relentlessly continued this narrow definition of what constitutes a bicycle to this day and has never been timid of throwing its weight around to enforce its singular will.

Some 60 years later, Scotland's Graeme Obree and his own interpretation of what constitutes a bicycle once again invoked the wrath of the UCI. Obree was born with a predisposition to be an outstanding athlete but, almost more importantly, to be able to think, engineer and improve human-to-machine solutions better than any athlete before or since. Obree's own struggles with the UCI from the outside seem to have a mythic David and Goliath quality.

In his competitive life, Obree broke three world records: in 1993, 1994 and 2013. And he was twice banned by the UCI for equipment violations. Faure and Mochet would certainly have empathised. Obree's most recent insights were to free his mind from Victorian constraints and to reimagine a machine that would perfectly express our bipedal potential, turn it though 90 degrees, and create a machine he could ride at 91km/h.

So why has the bicycle design survived, despite the UCI, if it's so bad? It's survived for nearly one hundred and fifty years, precisely because it's actually not that bad. In fact, it's reasonably good at low-to-moderate power outputs. We typically only use between 10 and 25 per cent of our theoretical maximum power when cycling. Most people ride most of the time at between 60 and 400 watts, which is a small fraction of what they are capable of as an explosive effort. And if we need to use short bursts of big power we tend to stand up on the pedals as if we're climbing stairs, or sprinting away from an attacking lion.

At Cyclefit, we often joke that we've spent the better part of our professional lives essentially fitting cavemen and women to a Victorian curiosity. By that we mean that our genome is substantially unchanged in 250,000 years, and bicycle dynamics are largely unchanged since the Boer War. Humans evolved to run and jump, not ride bikes – a self-evident fact of which we remind ourselves every day when we're working in our bike-fitting studios.

The butterfly effect

We wouldn't be having this conversation at all if nature hadn't failed to evolve a simple wheel and axle as a device to turn our 'potential' energy into usable 'kinetic' energy. Lean forward on the brow of a hill, and you can feel gravity acting on your mass, pulling you down. Now let's stand you on a skateboard and all of that potential is released in a satisfying kinetic rush. Nobody knows why nature failed to crack the evolution of the wheel across all those millions of years – one would have thought that radar for bats and sonar for dolphins was a bigger evolutionary step than a wheel and axle, but there we are. In fairness nature did evolve the eye on more than one occasion in multiple species.

We didn't get to a working wheel until around 5,000 years ago, and we were applying conscious thought, whereas nature was relying on the infinite blind maze of evolution, which requires billions of bad designs to get one good one. Nature can be partially forgiven.

Nature's failure to evolve a wheel meant that we needed to invent a device to make our walking bipedal biomechanics more efficient and sustainable. We wanted a machine to move our potential energy into sustainable kinetic energy, to release more speed and efficiency. The Victorians went off in two predominant directions, the penny-farthing and the modern safety bicycle – it was the BetaMax vs VHS, iPhone vs Android format war of the late 19th century. At least in this instance, the right design probably won, so we can at least be grateful we weren't left with the penny farthing as the dominant bicycle design – luckily the UCI wasn't created until 1900, so couldn't get involved in this debate! One can only imagine the carnage we could have now, commuting, racing and training on modern penny farthings – the NHS would be overwhelmed! I suspect that this could have happened had the UCI existed in 1890, and decreed for political reasons that the competition species of 'bicycle' had to look like a penny farthing, and the early manufacturers invested in it as the dominant design. This is known as 'path dependence', or the 'butterfly effect', whereby decisions that are made for social and political reasons have significant ramifications across the generations, which can be surprisingly difficult to reverse. Another example of this is the QWERTY keyboard I'm staring at hopelessly now, because I never learned to touch type. The QWERTY keyboard design, in an ironic twist, is a direct contemporary of the modern bicycle. It was devised by a Wisconsin newspaper editor and printer, Christopher Sholes, in the 1870s. The QWERTY design was an innovative solution intended to stop early typewriters getting stuck, as frequently used key bars clattered together. While this has had absolutely no relevance for at least the last 50 years, we continue to use the QWERTY layout on all of our devices – it's anachronistic and inefficient but, so far, has unwaveringly resisted revision from Apple, Microsoft, Google and others. A 150-year-old design, which made sense in a previous era, but which confoundingly persists to this day. Sound familiar? The QWERTY keyboard and bicycle are both flawed anachronisms that have so far resisted revision, largely for political, financial and cultural reasons.

We have to thank God that we were spared the penny farthing, though. As an aside, one of my most enigmatic clients was a penny farthing designer, builder and explorer called Joff. He came to see me almost 20 years ago after abandoning a round-the-world bike trip because he had started to get knee pain around Turkey, as I remember. My session with Joff made me review how the penny farthing riding position and biomechanics were driving his pain. Between us, we identified that his feet were too widely spaced on the pedals, which was driving an unnatural angle at the side of his knee. Joff remade the wheel and main axle himself (and may have even remade the entire bike). Problem solved and pain gone. He has traversed the globe on multiple occasions since on his self-made penny farthing, which he was kind enough to let me ride – which was enough to establish that unless you're Joff, a penny farthing is both daunting and inferior to a modern bicycle in every way (sorry, Joff).

The caveman and the Victorian contraption

So how does the 'modern' bicycle work with our midlife bodies – does it flatter or impede us? Are we in perfect harmony or in a continual tug of war with 19th-century biomechanics? To answer that question, we need to understand the physical proposition that the bicycle presents to our athletic form.

The closed kinetic chain

There's a raging (and perhaps irrelevant) debate in physio/orthopaedic circles, as to whether the cycling action is a closed kinetic chain (CKC) or open kinetic chain (OKC). A kinetic chain is simply all of the pivots and levers involved in one chain of movement – for example from the pelvis down to the toes on one leg, taking in the hip, knee and ankle joints on the way. In brief, because this can get tedious very quickly – the idea of kinetic chains being open or closed was introduced by Dr Arthur Steindler, an esteemed orthopaedic surgeon who worked in the US between the wars. Steindler's motivations were undoubtedly both intellectually lofty and clinically well-intended.

Here is what Steindler said: 'We designate an open kinetic chain a combination in which the terminal joint is free. A closed kinetic chain, on the other hand, is one in which the terminal joint meets with some considerable external resistance which prohibits or restrains its free motion'.

The terminal joint could be the hand throwing a javelin, or it can be the foot on a rotating pedal. It's the last joint in the sequence of moving segments that are forming the kinetic chain. Steindler wanted to draw a distinction between an open and closed chain because it's thought that the operation of the muscles is different from one environment to the other, and that this has clinical and rehabilitation implications. Part of this is down to the concept of proprioception – a person's perception of how nerves, muscles, bones, joints, tendons and ligaments are organised around a movement. Proprioception is key on a bicycle for a few reasons that can be distilled into one theme – cycling isn't a natural movement for our bodies to undertake and our own feedback is all too often counter-intuitive in this alien environment. After 20 years working with clients, Jules (Cyclefit co-founder) and I understand this and we're very careful about the questions we ask clients who are struggling with injury or underperformance, and how we weight their answers. For example, most clients don't know which leg is dominant in the pedal stroke (without a dual-side power meter). They will typically say, 'All my problems are on my right side, my left side is never a problem and is my good side, my left leg just gets on with it.' But this is what Jules and I hear: 'Your left leg is getting a free ride. Your right leg is actually better engaged, is being utilised more fully and is therefore more prone to over-use injury. And as a consequence what appears on your conscious radar is that your right leg is the good leg.'

We will then do some tests off the bike, such as partial single-leg squats – to review a client's proprioception off the bike, as well as to evaluate how torque is being applied to the crank through the pedal stroke, on the bike. From beginners to world champions, almost every rider finds it hard to form an accurate physical road map of what's going on when they ride. Including Jules and myself. Left to our own devices we would get everything wrong (and do). We need another person to be the dispassionate observer, measuring and crunching data. This is what we call Phil and Jules's Law – how it feels on a bicycle is almost never how it actually is on a bicycle.

Some have argued that since the pedal is rotating, then the foot is free and therefore cycling is open chain. The opposite also proves the point – when you run, the foot is acting against an unyielding ground, so the kinetic chain is closed. Our own experience is that cycling biomechanics are so wholly prescriptive and unusual that this effectively surpasses any notion of open or closed kinetic chains. Moreover, we view cycling as almost certainly a combination of open and closed chains, changing from one moment to the next.

In cycling, your foot is captured by a crank that rotates in a preordained circumference, which in turn closes your hip at the top of the pedal stroke, which acts upon a pelvis that is held by a saddle. Meanwhile, north of the border, you're leaning forwards on your hands, almost in a press-up position on the handlebars, loading your shoulders, with your spine flexed. Where exactly in the ancestral environment, or in nature, does that constitute a bipedal power posture? If you've ever felt like the bicycle is an alien spaceship, rather than a majestic translator of your human potential, then please instantly forgive yourself. There's no piece of sports equipment as potentially constricting as the humble bicycle (see chapter 5).

The physio's friend

So why, if cycling is biomechanically compromising or constraining, is the bike often the first line of defence for the medical profession, both as a rehab tool or as a migratory sport recommendation? Many of you reading this book will have transitioned to cycling from another sport – running, rugby, football, squash and hockey being the ones that readily spring to mind. In contrast, there are very few 50-year-old cyclists suddenly taking up rugby or hockey – this is almost exclusively a one-way street. The medical professional tends to love cycling for three predominant reasons. Firstly, because (theoretically) cycling should be a controlled and linear movement. Viewed from the front, the foot and knee ought to stay in line with the hip, specifically the anterior superior iliac spine (ASIS), throughout the pedalling movement. With all of the joints vertically stacked in alignment – hip, knee and ankle – there's minimal adverse lateral or torsional loading, so all of the joints are theoretically protected by the controlled motion. An example of this would be people who have injured their ACLs from skiing, rugby, football or squash. Some folk elect for reattachment surgery, in which case cycling may be a rehab tool. But some people decide to live their lives ACL-free, in which case cycling is both a rehab tool and a plausible final destination sport. Rugby and squash's loss is cycling's gain. Secondly, it is hypothetically possible to control joint loading forces precisely with cycling, for the very reason that hip and knee angles especially are being prescribed by the circumference of the pedal stroke. For example, we often work with clients who have had hip replacements or are recovering from serious hip injuries or surgery. Often, we're given a hip-in-flexion limitation to work with during the rehab phase. By adjusting the bike and crank positions we're able to precisely control the hip angle to keep the joint protected. However, not all surgeons or physios always understand that a client's natural ankle-movement patterning when pedalling will necessarily affect both the hip and the knee angles. For most people, the toes up/toes down (dorsiflexion/plantar flexion) patterning changes with both load and cadence. Thirdly – and we've all heard this one – cycling is 'non-impact', or at least it should be. My spine surgeon's rule that 'loaded bone is good bone' is pretty universal, but for some people the impact of full weight-bearing sport is just not recommended, or cannot be tolerated. We have many clients with a huge range of issues, where the impact of running or jumping is not advised in the short or long term – cartilage, ankle, hip, knee and spine injuries generally don't like high impacts. Cycling is one of a few activities that allows them to train as hard as they like and get a huge training effect, which has proven positive mental and physical benefits, but without imposing additional trauma onto their bodies.

The lack of trauma to bones, joints and muscles is one of the reasons cycling has also become the cross-training activity of choice for all sports. The central doctrine of structured training is predicated on gaining adaptive benefits from activity. The idea is that you deliberately stress the body outside of its current performance envelope to trigger an adaptive response to create more strength and resilience – building brick on brick. But an activity like running (especially sprinting) creates a relatively high degree of micro-trauma to the muscles, a temporary scarring within the muscle structure itself. A sensible and well-conditioned athlete can actually use cycling as a way to get a big cardiovascular dividend on their non-running days, while still allowing the muscles to adapt. Moreover, if the cycling session isn't too onerous they can reasonably expect increased muscle adaption due to increased blood flow through the capillaries (small blood vessels). And obviously, at some point, they will inevitably work out that cycling is a lot more fun than running. I run 5km once or twice a week – partly because it's short and fits into family life, but also because I know that in my late 50s it's very good for both bone density and sarcopenia. I make a point of only ever running off-road on trails and tracks, to minimise impact and joint loading forces, but also because the uneven surface enhances stabilisation muscle engagement. I use an appropriate shoe for my wide and high volume foot (Mizuno Wave) and a podiatrist-prescribed running orthotic. I'm conscious of my running style – my podiatrist recommends I decrease stride length and increase cadence. And I stretch both before and after. And yet despite all of this, when I get back from running, I feel aches and pains in so many areas – glutes, hamstrings, calves, quads and my right Achilles. Running may be good for me but it also comes at a price. There's simply no way I could run every day in the same way that, fitness permitting, it's possible to cycle every day. And that, of course, is the point – cycling should be minimally impactive on your bones, muscles and tendons but as maximally impactive on your cardio system as you care to make it.

Confounding variables

For some people, the bicycle is their virtual second home – they can eat and put on a rain jacket – all without stopping. They can ride all day, train as much as they like, never get injured or sore. When they ride, they have a fluidity and ease of motion that's almost poetic – us old-timers used to call it 'souplesse'. They often look better on the bike than they do off it.

Twenty years ago, at a charity ride in Devon, I met a former pro who had ridden in the Tour de France in the 1960s. I was introduced to this slight and stooped ageing gentleman before the ride – he had a pronounced limp as he walked, and one shoulder was distinctly lower than the other. I was still racing regularly and was probably the fittest and strongest I have ever been. After about 50km we hit the big climbs going up onto Exmoor, and the racers pulled away from the more fitness-orientated riders and families. A group of about six went of us went over the climb and naturally moved into an alternating paceline as we headed into a powerful headwind. As an old racer I quite automatically evaluate any group I'm riding with – technique, physique, road craft, intelligence. I can't help myself. Road racing is like a three-dimensional game of chess where we all seek to share, and then exploit, each other's strengths and weaknesses – the ruthless mechanics of cooperate v defect played out on tarmac. This wasn't a road race and there was to be no official winner, but I still went through the critical assessment process anyway. Only one rider stood out in this group as being in any way particularly special – he was always in the right place in the paceline, accelerated gently and assertively when he needed to, had superb biomechanics and exuded poise and balance on the bike. As we descended into the valley, I took his wheel on trust without touching our brakes at all. Looking back, I saw fresh air and a deserted road. We started the next climb side by side at a pace we both knew was on the brisk side of acceptable. He then tapped me on the elbow and took a piece of pre-buttered malt loaf out of a some tin foil and handed it to me. It was only then that I looked into the face of my new riding partner – Colin, the 1960s Tour rider – a man twice my age and alive to his natural environment. The next 100km were an education I'll never forget – the slightly crooked, hunched and gracefully ageing gentleman had metamorphosed into a phenominal athlete of rare elegance and economy of movement. The bike is a complex and demanding instrument that flatters particular, and sometimes peculiar, morphology and psychology. It was a valuable lesson, both as a racer and as a bike-fitter, that I have never forgotten. It should be said that I struggled to keep up with Colin when he was already over 60 years of age. Had he been closer to my age, then he would have left me gasping and unable to stay on his wheel.

At the other end of the spectrum from Colin are folk who never truly feel comfortable, efficient or powerful on a bike. The most common feedback we hear is that it is impossible for them to express their potential within the confines of a bicycle. Over the years we've worked with riders at every waypoint on this spectrum. Sometimes they are the same rider, who travel from one end of the scale to the other, due to injury, illness and weight gain/loss for example, and then back again. But what is it that defines one group relative to the other? And how do some sportsmen and women migrate to cycling with alarming alacrity, moving from the fast lane in their previous sport straight into the fast lane in cycling? And how do others bring all the physical condition and competition ethic that comes from elite sport and yet struggle to feel effective on a bike, and consistently fail to achieve the results or fitness they desire?

The prescriptive abstract environment

The bicycle is ultimately prescriptive because every part of your body is constrained – the saddle by the pelvis, the foot by the pedal and your upper body through the connection to the handlebars. Forget the question as to whether cycling is an open or closed chain because all the links in the chain are fundamentally connected and therefore exert an influence upon each other. This can be positive and negative – positive in the sense that when you stand and pedal at low cadence (for example, going up a steep hill) with very high force, you're bracing the high torque being generated through your powerful glutes, quads and calves against your upper body, as if you're pulling on a tight wellington boot. There's no way you could do it without pushing with your legs and pulling with your arms. You're effectively and deliberately 'associating' your upper body with your lower body. But this is frequently problematic, because your body will unconsciously adapt around an instability or asymmetry, which over time can result in pain or injury. For example, an instability in the foot can sometimes lead to a poorly tracking knee and hip, all the way through to the upper body and into the shoulder, arm and hand. This unusual connection of underlying cause to distant physical manifestation is inherently less likely with running or walking, where your body has almost total freedom to move and compensate (we'll come back to this).

When you run, you're choosing the length of every single step in response to the terrain, with your pelvis free to adapt to your gait changes.

There's little doubt that the bicycle is an innately abstract environment for your body. There aren't many sports or athletic pastimes that you conduct sitting down with a flexed spine and flexed hip, trying to produce high amounts of torque and power – rowing being the other obvious one. The abstraction is further exacerbated due to a lack of direct ground contact. We evolved to mostly function in direct relationship to the ground – we spring off our toes when we run, utilising our strong glute, quad and calf extensor muscles to bounce away from the ground and onto the next step. None of this happens in cycling, your relationship to the earth is different – you're umbilically attached to a machine, feeling your way around the world via two rotating gyroscopes and a couple of centimetres of rubber.

This level of abstraction may partially explain why rowers tend to transition to cycling faster than any other group of elite sports people. Aside from their well-adapted cardiovascular system, horsepower and training ethic, rowers are also used to being imprisoned by a machine with no ground contact. It takes them seconds to flick the mental switch from making a boat move quickly in water to making a bike move quickly through the air. It appears to be instantaneous, most especially with lightweight scullers.

In contrast, it would be easy to assume that distance runners will seamlessly transition from running on the track or trail to running on a bike. They are generally light, well-conditioned and have a superb training ethic, but runners also often fail to adapt as quickly to high-level cycling and struggle to feel as natural producing power on a bike as they do running in the hills or on a track. My own view is that one of the biggest contributors to their initial feelings of discombobulation is that they are unconscious freedom junkies. They don't like to be constrained by a machine and they don't want their feet held in pedals turning in prescribed circles. And, most importantly, when they toe-off they don't really want the ground to go with them, as happens with the pedal. This foot–pedal relationship, which is the immoveable rock and architectural set-in point for successful cycling, is often an anathema to runners when they first start cycling. When I evaluate runners who are having problems with injury or performance, it's the simple dynamics of pedalling that they frequently struggle with – it's like they're trying to shake their foot free of the pedal on every stroke. They are leaking power and efficiency at the connection of the foot–pedal interface because of an unconscious and unwanted physical adaptation that comes with being permanently connected. The first step is often getting them to try emulating some of the freedom of running which is so familiar to them. We do that by getting them to cycle in their running shoes on flat pedals. The reaction is often revelatory – their pedalling and torque application transforms, and as a consequence their perception of the process improves. We go into the details of how best to marry bikes to riders in chapter 5.

The hypermobile v stiff – micro v macro spectrum

Our friend and collaborator Alex Fugallo, who is an osteopath, introduced us to a flexibility spectrum that he uses to triage his patients, which we've also found useful to contextualise our clients and work out how we can best help them. Alex uses a functional movement screen to review and record his patients' general and specific levels of flexibility (we use our own cycling-specific method). At one end of the spectrum there are people who are hypermobile and at the other end, those who have the least range of motion in their muscles and joints. Most of us, of course, sit somewhere in the middle of the bell curve and are not outliers towards the extreme poles. The point being that those of us who are hypermobile have different issues compared to those who are challenged by range-of-motion issues – a euphemism for stiff as a board. Hypermobile individuals can struggle with sufficient strength to control their excessive range of movement – they often struggle to find their happy place and constantly look for joint end-of-range to feel physically controlled, anchored and calm. We often see them sit on the bike with an exaggerated lumbar lordosis – i.e. the opposite of a slouch and with locked elbows to try to fix themselves into a stable posture. At the other end of the spectrum, athletes who lack flexibility often find that their flexibility deficit is pulling them into biomechanically poor positions that expose them to injury and pain. We frequently see their pelvises being pulled back (into a slouch) by tight hamstrings, or their knees driven out by poor hip-in-flexion range (see chapter 5). It makes sense that the advice given to both parties is different, quite aside from the bike fit ramifications. Alex Fugallo, somewhat controversially, explains: 'Does a hypermobile person really need any more range of motion? Should they actually be stretching a great deal, when what they really need is strength? Conversely, do we necessarily need a very stiff person to be any stronger before they can significantly increase their ranges of motion?'

Our colleague Phil Burt, ex-lead physio and bike fitter for Team GB, introduced a wonderful contextual background to Alex's approach at the 2012 International Cyclefit Conference (ICS). Phil pioneered his own way of internally triaging his clients as being on a micro-adjuster–macro-absorber spectrum. The micro-adjusters are the ones who occupy most bike fitters' and physios' time. They are 'the princesses and the peas' of the cycling community, at both amateur and professional levels. Micro-adjusters adapt very poorly to any change in themselves (such as injury or illness), or misalignment in their equipment set-up. It could be that a cleat has moved or a saddle has slipped a millimetre or two. Not only will they feel it but they are also more likely to get physical pain, and even anxiety, as a consequence. Micro-adjusters, by definition, have to be obsessional perfectionists to function consistently at a good level. Micro-adjusters are great clients to work with from our perspective – they are impressively engaged in the process, we see them a lot, they give instant feedback, they generally have superb insight into their own bodies, they work us hard and so we also learn a lot, and best of all, they all do their homework! Micro-adjusters literally keep us all in business, and we tend to form the closest working relationships with them.

At the other end of the spectrum are pure macro-absorbers – nothing hurts, nothing bothers them, they unconsciously ride around any problem that comes their way. You can quite literally give them the wrong bike off the team truck and they may never know (real example by the way of a well-known Tour de France winner). We tend to see macro-absorbers much less often. On a pro level, we only see them at team camps, if they are changing bike or shoe sponsor and need to be set up again, or if they have a big crash and injury and suddenly find that they don't macro-absorb anymore.

If we combine Alex's mobility spectrum with Phil's micro v macro spectrum, what can we conclude? It's way too simplistic to think that macro-absorbers are the hypermobiles and micros are the stiffest athletes. That actually doesn't fit our experience of what we see at all, with either amateur or professional riders. Micro-adjusters, we suggest, are most likely to hang out at either ends of the spectrum – very stiff or very mobile. And macro-absorbers are arguably most likely to be the ones right in the middle of the bell curve, having an optimal cocktail of strength and flexibility.

By the way, a quick thought experiment – where do you think you sit on both spectrums? Do you tend to be a micro-adjuster or a macro-absorber? And do you view yourself as a generally mobile person or tending to be stiff and lacking in range? This may help you contextualise your own experience and physical trajectory as a midlife athlete. Personally, I think I used to be predominantly a macro-absorber and more towards the flexible end of the spectrum. As a racer I didn't have too many injuries and ironically, full disclosure, thought very little about my position on the bike from season to season. Until, that is, I had a serious crash and fractured my spine, which required spine-fusion surgery. In an instant I went right up to the micro-adjusting end of the spectrum, where I'll probably always reside. At least I know. I have to do my homework if I want stay functional and riding. By the way, flexibility and strength are two very important components of bike tolerance and resilience, but there are many others that we'll look at in chapter 5 — foot structure and posture, and pelvis architecture being two of the most important.

One of the guiding predicates of this book is that the bicycle is actually an abstract and alien environment for human beings, whatever the benign intentions of our Victorian ancestors. We mostly don't question the fact that the modern bicycles we ride today are almost identical in architecture, dimension and biomechanical interface to something that was designed around the same time as the Gunfight at the O.K. Corral. For most of us, most of the time, the bicycle is luckily just good enough, achieves what we need and doesn't hurt or injure us. But there's simply no device or piece of equipment in the world which has such a complete and dictatorial conjunction with our bodies. Our feet are trapped by the pedals and our pelvis held in position by the saddle, while we lean forward at an acute angle to fix our hands on the handlebars. And we're then expected to exert ourselves over a protracted period to our theoretical maximum. It's a more challenging proposition than most of us assume and needs to be regularly assessed as we age and demand more performance from our bodies. It's the job of this book to evaluate the challenges and suggest strategies to optimise your connection to this bizarre contraption, which we've largely accepted as the norm since we were kids and wobbled down the road on our first flight. Whatever the history and underpinnings, the bicycle now exists as an identifiable frame of reference. And despite, or maybe even because of, murky politics, the bicycle is loved by many in its present form. To tell the whole truth, it's also loved by us at Cyclefit. We're as sentimentally and romantically connected to the seven strangely arranged tubes as any fan or enthusiast. The only difference is that we're also alive to all the pitfalls and challenges that await us if we take it for granted.

3

WILL I DIE?

Whether you or I will die if we cycle into and beyond middle age is, of course, a deliberately glib and simplistic question, which deserves fleshing out a little, while we still can. Firstly, we're not particularly interested in the likelihood of death caused by traffic accidents or self-inflicted trauma caused by falling off our bikes. In fact, only 99 cyclists were killed in road accidents in 2018, and the number has remained relatively stable since. Although one death is one too many, as a proportion of the level of cycling participation across all activities – commuting, racing and training – this number is statistically very low. There were 4205 KSIs (killed or seriously injured) cycling incidents in the same period, which accounted for a relatively higher 14 per cent of all road incidents across all modalities. Statistically therefore, we only have a vanishingly small chance of being involved in an accident that's going to kill us, and only a slightly higher chance of a serious injury.

Enough about accidents for the moment – we are focussing in this chapter on the chances of cycling actually contributing to, or even triggering, a fatal medical event and upon the modifiable factors and behaviours we can influence, which will help ameliorate our risks. That is to say, can cycling actually be a driver of increasing our risk of serious health problems and, if so, what are the best clinically proven measures that we can take to protect ourselves? And does the evidence show that the perceived risk (and therefore preventative measures) are the same for men and women? Of all the possible fatal events our imagination can conjure, the most frightening must be a heart-related incident. Are they the metaphorical shark circling in the water for all of us when we push the intensity/duration mix to the outside of our theoretical envelope?

Let's therefore look at some very specific facts around participation in high-intensity events and likelihood of death. One of the best-known endurance events in the UK is Ride London, which shared its data with us, collated over seven events since 2013. A massive 179,500 participants have taken part, with an average age of 45, riding all the available distances, giving an average of 130km per person. This equates to a collective distance of 23 million kilometres. To date, only six people have died – one from a head injury caused by a crash, and five more due to heart attacks. You can numerically interpret these numbers in many ways, so here are just a few. There's a fatal cardiac event every 5 million kilometres pedalled or there is a 1:36,000 chance of dying if you ride the event, which is of course tiny. And there's even less risk if you're a woman because even though women make up nearly 35 per cent of the total number of riders, there haven't (to date) been any female fatalities. This is a theme that pervades this chapter, in that female veteran athletes are reassuringly dull when it comes to adverse heart issues. There's no way to make this sound any more exciting – any midlife female athlete having a cardiovascular event around excess exercise is a complete statistical outlier.

Cardiologists like binary

It takes a special kind of doctor to be able to operate on their fellow human being's heart. At its most extreme, some heart surgeons will have the opportunity to look down at a patient's empty chest cavity after removing their heart, before refilling the space with a transplanted organ. Consequently, cardiologists seek, crave and venerate cause and effect certainty. Patients want the same – we all want a diagnostic procedure, with a clear result, followed by a predictable treatment path.

Clinician and patient are mutually invested in confidence, belief and certitude – after all, this is heart surgery, not fixing tennis elbow. Except, as we have seen, midlife athletes are the pathfinders in terms of exercise dosing when it comes to the veteran athlete heart. We're the real-world crash-test dummies, who are now the subjects of contemporary 10- and 20-year longitudinal studies that will give us clear answers to fundamental questions which right now are still frustratingly unknown. For example:

- Is there a correlation between exercise duration and intensity, and cardiac damage?
- What is the optimal exercise dose for midlife cyclists to balance performance and health?
- Does the exercise dose/intensity recommendation differ for male and female veteran athletes?
- What are the modifiable factors that can improve health and performance outcomes for veteran athletes?

Answers to these questions will be substantially known in a couple of decades thanks to the research that is being currently undertaken, but for the moment we consulted with two treating consultant cardiologists – Dr Stephens and Dr Audrius Simiatis, both self-confessed immoderate midlife cyclists. And also with eminent cardiac researchers – Dr Ahmed Merghani and Dr Gemma Parry-Williams, both younger and more moderate exercisers. Drs Merghani and Parry-Williams are running precisely the kind of research studies that will yield the clarity and direction which veteran athletes crave. All four doctors were generous, patient and clear-eyed about what they knew and what they didn't.

Lord save us from moderation

Moderation in everything is apparently good for us. It's screamed at us from every health guideline and evangelising headline, covering everything from alcohol consumption, to exercise, to calorie consumption. And when it comes to exercise and cycling, moderation is unquestionably beneficial when juxtaposed to non-participation. Fairly small doses of exercise (the UK government recommends 150 minutes of 'moderate' or 75 minutes of 'vigorous' exercise per week) stimulate a veritable barrage of well-documented and wholly positive and powerful effects: 40 per cent less chance of Type II diabetes, 35–50 per cent less chance of cardiovascular (CV) disease, 20 per cent less chance of cancer risk, 25–30 per cent less risk of a stroke, as well as reduced blood pressure, lower body weight and lower cholesterol and so on. The overall picture is a healthy sunlit upland of marvellousness. Not only that, but we'll be in a better mental state to enjoy this new health landscape for longer: we'll be less depressed, cognitively rejuvenated and better protected against dementia; recent studies show that physical exercise is one of the most powerful modifiable factors in the personal fight against Alzheimer's.

The list of potential benefits of moderate exercise is so long it's best measured in furlongs and is growing all the time, verified by a huge body of research – James H. O'Keefe et al. express it with this thought: 'Physical exercise, though not a drug, possesses many traits of a powerful pharmacological agent.' In their research paper, they question whether there may be an optimal dosing load, which we would be unwise to exceed. All roads lead to moderation. There is little contention surrounding the benefits of moderate exercise, other than what 'moderate' constitutes. In fact, the word 'moderate' has been so ubiquitously and routinely used by everyone from the NHS to tabloid scaremongering articles that the term contributes little to informed exercise discussion.

A life less moderate

But this book isn't really aimed at those who seek to be moderate. In point of fact, if you seek moderation you may not need this book at all – stick to 14 units of alcohol a week, eat a varied diet, do 30–60 minutes of moderate to vigorous exercise per day a few times per week, and go to the occasional challenging yoga class, and a whole universe of uncontested positivity is almost certainly guaranteed, with no known adverse side effects.

But where is the fun in that? Many of us seek to be immoderate because it's intrinsically more involving and challenging. For the purposes of this chapter we're not particularly interested in moderate training or exercise, mostly because it's entirely uncontroversial.

Do more, die less?

The positive effects of exercise upon coronary heart disease (CHD) were first statistically evaluated in the late 1940s by Dr Jerry Morris, and his pioneering study that compared 31,000 sedentary tram and bus drivers with their comparatively active conductor co-workers. The latter, Morris worked out, climbed between 500 and 750 steps per day on their trams and buses, whereas the drivers sat firmly on their backsides for almost all of the day. A perfect control and study group. Both groups pretty much shared the same diet, background, income, education and lifestyle. They were demarcated by only one significant variable – the drivers were extremely sedentary and the conductors were early forerunners of the now ubiquitous 10,000 steps regime, by climbing up and down flights of stairs every day of their working lives. It was a point of single binary distinction between two almost congruent groups, and a piece of lateral genius to put them at the centre of a heart study. Morris found that the conductors not only had almost 50 per cent less incidence of CHD (coronary heart disease) than the drivers, but if the conductors did get CHD it was of a more benign nature and generally later in their life. The headline figure was that the conductors were half as likely to die prematurely than the drivers. The conclusion of this highly reputable and ground-breaking epidemiological study was that 'physically active work' gave a tangible and highly protective effect against CHD and its natural corollary of early death.

It should be mentioned that this revolutionary study was not in any way trivial. Many at the time thought that exercise was innately harmful in the long term. In the same way that driving a car for thousands of miles would wear the components to eventual failure, so running or walking or physical labour would wear out your joints and body parts over time. Not much was known about stressing the body to create adaptive resilience to bigger physical loads in the future. This study indicated that it was exercise alone which was responsible for the positive causative structural changes in the body. It was the exercise that was positively remodelling the heart over time.

Morris went a step further with a study published in 1973, which looked at 17,000 middle-aged but sedentary civil servants between the ages of 40 and 64. Morris was interested in how their structured external leisure activities, outside work, would affect their future cardiac health and risk. The benefit of this study was its ability to look at different exercise profiles and the statistical outcomes. Is badminton better for you than bridge? Is playing football or running better for you than table tennis? The findings gave more granular detail than the original conductor/driver study and produced a huge amount of data, but the headline was very simple and best summed up by Morris himself: 'Vigorous exercise is a natural defence of the body, with a protective effect on the ageing heart against ischemia [decreased blood flow and oxygen] and its consequences.'

For the study, vigorous exercise was defined as having a peak energy output of 7.5kcal per minute, or 450kcal per hour. That isn't vigorous at all compared to climbing Alpe d'Huez, where a 50-year-old cyclist might work at a rate of 1000kcal per hour.

Nevertheless, the trend seemed clear – activity and exercise increased cardiovascular health and reduced CHD. And the more you exercised, at a more vigorous rate, the more you could reduce CHD risk into and beyond middle age.

This goes back to our discussion about evolutionary irrelevance – it only took 250,00 years of being a modern human being to arrive at an epiphany in the 1970s (well within the memorable lifetime of most of us) to understand the true link between the protective effect of exercise and cardiac health into middle age and beyond. We managed to prove the world was round in 1492, but it was to take nearly another 500 years to establish how to reduce coronary heart disease. In mitigation, as we now know, it wasn't until the last hundred years that people lived long enough in statistical terms to actually suffer heart disease – until almost the end of the 19th century, the average European died before their 35th birthday.

The unworried unwell

The 'do more, die less' view orthodoxy prevailed through the 1970s and into the early 1980s, and was typified by Jim Fixx, author of *The Complete Running Book*. Jim Fixx was the ultimate midlife runner and father of the modern jogging /running movement. It's probably true to say that Nike and Adidas owed, and maybe even still owe, much of their share price to Mr Fixx.

Jim Fixx started running in 1967, at the age of 35. At the time he weighed 97kg and had smoked 40 cigarettes a day for many years. When he died, running alone in Vermont in 1984, aged 52, he weighed around 70kg and hadn't smoked a cigarette in nearly two decades. The autopsy showed that Jim Fixx had suffered a fatal heart attack due to atherosclerosis of his coronary arteries – one of them was 95 per cent blocked. We'll talk much more about atherosclerosis vascular disease (ASVD) in this chapter and learn that not all ASVD is created equal.

Jim Foxx's dreadfully ironic and iconic death polarised people at the time according to individual cognitive bias. To the millions of runners he mobilised in the US and all over the world it was a tragedy, but at least he died doing what he loved and in the finest form of his life. Moreover it was quickly hypothecated that running probably elongated his life to 52, given that his father, Calvin Fixx, died at the age of 43 after two heart attacks – the second of which was fatal.

To Fixx's critics it was the end of do more, die less. He was one of the fittest middle-aged men in the world but still managed to die at the same average age of someone living in the US in the 1920s. Jim Fixx became an easy target for the detractors of the emerging exercise revolution – it was elementary that running too much had killed him or, at the very least, tangibly contributed to his death. To many people, Jim Fixx's premature death proved, in the most public and spectacular way possible, that Dr Morris was either wrong or, at least, not entirely right to believe that vigorous exercise has a natural and protective defence on the ageing heart. Or, at least, that this was not necessarily a biological universal law. It's possible to fill an entire book on this fascinating subject alone, but for our own purposes it's worth teasing out a couple of themes. Firstly, Dr Morris was looking at sample sizes of 17,000 people whereas Jim Fixx was a sample size of precisely one, however fascinating and seemingly contradictory his sample size appears. Secondly, it's entirely possible that Jim Fixx could have under-survived even his father had he continued on his mid-1960s life path (see Dr Stephens' comments below). Thirdly, we'll never know if Jim Fixx experienced prior to his death any symptoms that he ignored, or even if he could have been a little more diligent in terms of his own cardiac screening and testing, given his family history. We'll talk later about QRISK scoring, but one of the first questions all these risk calculators ask is whether you have a parent who suffered from heart disease under the age of 60.

Leaving aside for one moment, expensive and often invasive testing, simply joining elementary dots can be the most powerful form of screening. Jim Fixx was a member of Mensa, the high-IQ society, and an intelligent thinker. Maybe he didn't look under this particular cardiac health stone because he didn't want to know what was under it.

Dr Parry-Williams speculates that athletes sometimes, consciously or unconsciously, hide their symptoms. Maybe the feeling of ischemia (lack of oxygen to the heart muscle) is just an assumed part of the feeling of training and racing at a high level? Jim Fixx may have been acclimatised, or even addicted to, that feeling of anaerobic deficit which is an intrinsic part of interval training? Anaerobic literally means 'occurring, or existing, in the absence of free oxygen'. Anaerobic activity occurs right at the top 10 per cent of our exercise spectrum capability, long after oxygen has been abandoned by the body as a dominant metabolite. In that sense, anaerobic and ischemia are close hypoxic cousins because they are twin states of being which are devoid of oxygen. Athletes who train regularly at an intense level are compelled to 'make friends' with this kind of deficit or pain. This may contain a small risk to a veteran athlete who has an underlying propensity for heart disease, but arguably also familiarises our body's cardiovascular system for the onslaught of being oxygen deprived. Maybe Jim Fixx just missed the early signs? Or maybe he had created a new category of the 'unworried unwell', as opposed to the more normal 'worried well' who routinely fill doctors' surgeries? That is, of course, highly speculative on my part. We approached Dr Stephens for his comment on Jim Fixx's early death. 'Jim Fixx is where evidence and anecdote collide. Exercise isn't a panacea, but neither does it cause cardiovascular disease nor sudden death. Jim Fixx died 10 years later than his father. His genetic background was very adverse. He had smoked and came to sport late. I suspect running gave him seven more years of life.'

The 'Lancification' of cycling

If Jim Fixx was the paradigm-shifting running evangelist responsible for mobilising a generation into vigorous and structured exercise, then I suggest that Lance Armstrong was cycling's catalysing force in the late 1990s and all through the 2000s. Until that time, competitive cycling, at least in the UK and US, was a comparatively niche activity. And those of us who transacted the business of road racing and time trialling around remote country roads at dawn were considered extreme and possibly a little strange. Things changed when Lance Armstrong published his book, *It's Not About The Bike*, in 2000. At the time of publication, Armstrong had recently beaten cancer against overwhelming odds. He was a genuine medical miracle who went from deathbed back to professional cycling in just over two years. Lance went on to win the Tour de France in 1999. Notwithstanding the controversy that was to follow, this was at the time an incredible story of courage and renewal. Personally I think that revisionist history will be somewhat kinder to Armstrong, with respect to the transformational effect he had in both the cancer community and how he revolutionised cycling participation across the globe.

Our client base at Cyclefit changed almost overnight, from competitive men and women seeking speed and injury solutions to a slightly older male and female demographic who had been motivated into action by Armstrong's story. Some folk would come into their initial Cyclefit session clutching a copy of *It's Not About The Bike* and talk about a relative or friend who was engaged in a personal battle with cancer. Sometimes it was the person themselves who was living with cancer and wanted to, just like Armstrong, make the bike part of their personal arsenal. Armstrong even influenced oncologists who questioned whether vigorous exercise, in the form of cycling, could contribute to active cancer therapy.

It was a remarkable revolution for recreational cycling all over the world. And it introduced new challenges and questions. Our average client became a middle-aged man or women, who was either coming from a sedentary background or migrating from another sport. They were armed with the Armstrong-focussed zealotry of a convert, and the noble goal of riding a mountain stage in the Tour de France, called L'Étape du Tour. We quickly learned that most of these midlifers would not only achieve their immediate goal but go on to make high intensity training part of their life. They set even bolder plans and objectives to achieve on their bikes – La Marmotte (the huge one-day Alpine event), Haute Routes and multi-day events in the mountains became de rigueur for a new generation for whom Armstrong, almost single-handedly, switched on the biking gene. Often the Armstrong disciples would go on to positively enthuse their own friends and family to create a second generation of midlifers – it was like a positive pyramid scheme where everyone would switch on their own peer group to the excitement and adventure of intense cycling. It was a very exciting and hugely satisfying time to be involved with cycling.

But let's get back to the public health context of all these midlife cyclists out there in the mountains pushing their bodies to their limits and deliberately not being moderate in any known sense of the word. I think most of us participating in high-intensity cycling self-selected into the prevailing view that Jim Fixx was anomalous and in no way presaged a new orthodoxy that viewed vigorous exercise as potentially damaging to middle-aged athletes. Well, I did.

Structural changes study

A benign tension of cognitive bias around veteran heart health continued until recently. Those of us personally invested in middle-aged performance dissembled around a somewhat vague but comforting 'overall benefit' perspective. On the other side of the argument were some of the press, and even some other publications who should know better, who periodically aimed at the same bullseye: 'Too much exercise will kill you!'

What was needed was the blinding light of objective medical scientific research to cut through the comparative collective ignorance on the subject of structural changes in the heart, as a response to increased training loads in veteran male and female cyclists and runners. Step up Dr Merghani and his associates Aneil Malhotra and Sanjay Sharma, in a 2012 study for the Department of Cardiovascular Sciences, St George's, University of London.

The Merghani study ran for three years between 2012 and 2015, specifically to look at the possibility of exercise-induced heart remodelling. But Merghani, in his own words, was also more generally interested in assessing the 'emerging number of reports suggesting that intense exercise may have an adverse impact on an otherwise normal heart, and review the morbidity and mortality associated with sport, and pose the question whether one can have too much of a good thing.'

The Merghani study recruited 152 veteran runners and cyclists, all over 40, with an average age of 51 (+/-9 years), all defined as lifelong heavy exercisers, having trained for an average of 31 years (+/-12.6 years). By the way, the study group also contained 16 national champions and five world champions, 70 per cent of whom were male and 30 per cent female. All exercised for at least eight hours every week. None of the group smoked or had previously displayed any symptoms of heart disease or cardiac disturbance. Merghani/Malhotra/Sharma also ran a control group of 92 sedentary and moderate exercisers (exercising less than five hours per week) – individuals with a mean age of 52.5 (+/-5.4 years), of which 47 were female.

The study and control groups both underwent intensive diagnostic testing, including echocardiograms, cardiopulmonary testing, electrocardiograms (ECGs), cardiac magnetic resonance imaging (MRI), coronary computerised tomography (CT) scans and Holter 24-hour heart monitoring, among other assessments. These tests represent the current gold standard in cardiac examinations. Somewhat surprisingly, the control and study groups had very similar blood pressure scores, 123.6 and 125.6 mm Hg (blood pressure is measured in millimeteres of mercury – mm HG) and also shared very congruent total cholesterol scores (4.42 and 4.52) mmol/l stands (millimoles per litre). But there was a predictably huge discrepancy in the two groups' VO_2 Max – the sedentary control group posted an average of 27.9 mL/kg/min but the athlete group averaged over 60 per cent more at 43.3 mL/kg/min!

Merghani et al. published their revelatory study in 2017 to an intellectually engaged but nevertheless shocked medical community. However, an unintended consequence of the study was that it also re-energised the reductive populist press about why too much exercise could be bad for you.

At this point it's worth mentioning that Dr Merghani, who generously gave up his time during the research of this book, is an endlessly patient and serious research cardiologist. He's also, despite some of the prima facie nature of some of his research (see later in this chapter), a wholehearted supporter of the positive effects of lifelong exercise. He remarked: 'The benefits of exercise are irrefutable. Individuals engaging in regular exercise have a favourable cardiovascular risk profile for coronary artery disease and reduce their risk of myocardial infarction by 50 per cent. Exercise promotes longevity of life, reduces the risk of some malignancies, retards the onset of dementia, and is considered an antidepressant.'

The first revelation of the study was that the athlete group had a significantly higher incidence of 'arrhythmias' compared to the control sedentary group. An arrhythmia is an inconsistency in the rhythm of your heartbeat – it can be too fast (tachycardia) or too slow (bradycardia), or you may exhibit uneven or missed heartbeat.

The athlete group had a much higher incidence of all types of arrhythmias compared to the sedentary (or moderate exercise) control group. Eleven per cent of the athlete group had supraventricular tachycardia (SVT), while six per cent of the athlete group had largely nocturnal pauses in their heartbeats of more than 2.5 seconds (including me) compared to zero in the control group. About 4 per cent of the athlete group exhibited atrial flutter (AF) compared to zero for the control group. While SVT, pauses in heartbeats and AF are all deemed to be largely benign arrythmias, it's certainly interesting that all these symptoms were markedly more prevalent in the athlete group than in the control group. Interesting, but not necessarily worrying.

But there was a slightly more worrying finding in relation to a particular type of arrhythmia called non-sustained ventricular tachycardia (NSVT, or sometimes just VT). NSVT is a short period of faster heartbeats – at least 120 beats per minute (bpm) – which lasts for less than 30 seconds but for more than three successive beats. Often NSVT happens under our conscious radar – it's picked up only by extended ECGs, measured in this instance using the 24-hour Holter test. None of the sedentary group exhibited any NSVT, but eight per cent of the athlete group displayed significant NSVT – and all of them were male subjects. An example finding was a 52-year-old male cyclist who had a 14-beat run of NSVT but was totally asymptomatic. Many cardiologists would nevertheless err on the side of caution and fit an implantable cardioverter defibrillator (ICD) into this particular individual, to prevent a sudden cardiac event.

But the context is more nuanced, as seven per cent of the athlete cohort team exhibited similar symptoms – so do we install an ICD into all of them or indeed every male veteran athlete just to be sure? Is an ICD, or even a pacemaker, the new normal of being a high-level veteran athlete pushing the body beyond its evolutionary design life? The prevalence of these NSVTs in the veteran athlete group, where there were none in the control group – who, to reiterate, were either sedentary or exercising in a moderate fashion (under five hours per week) – was a completely new finding. The incidence of NSVTs in the athlete group was a concern, not only because these arrhythmias can be intrinsically sinister themselves, but they may also presage other conditions and risks such as:

- Atherosclerosis (coronary heart disease, or CHD)
- Myocardial fibrosis
- Inflammation

Let's break down these three issues down a little further.

The terms atherosclerosis and coronary heart disease (CHD) are, confusingly, often used interchangeably. But whatever nomenclature we choose to use, the set of symptoms both these terms describe are vitally important because over 80 per cent of sudden deaths in veteran athletes are attributable to CHD. What this means is that although we may have only about a 1:50,000 chance of dying as a veteran athlete in an endurance event such as the London Marathon or Ride 100, if we do succumb to more strenuous efforts than our ageing bodies can endure, there's a greater than 80 per cent chance that the cause will be linked in some way to CHD.

Atherosclerosis is a somewhat all-encompassing title for 'plaques', or deposits that build up in our coronary (heart) arteries. These plaques can comprise fat, cholesterol, calcium and more fibrous material, or any combination of these ingredients. Clinically, atherosclerosis is split into one of three categories:

1 Soft plaques – fatty, unstable and inflamed plaque deposits.
2 Calcified plaques – these are more stable and harder deposits.
3 Mixed morphology – these plaques comprise a mixture of calcium, fatty and fibrous material and are felt to be the most unstable of all.

A heart attack (or myocardial infarction) occurs when these plaques rupture and then clots or thromboses cause a blockage in the coronary arterial flow itself. CHD is the great white shark that haunts the dreams of middle-aged men everywhere – I say men because so many of the causes and symptoms of heart disease don't seem to apply on either a statistical or anecdotal basis to female veteran athletes. According to Dr Parry-Williams, 'It's very rare for women to succumb to sudden death in sport.' And from the clinical frontline dealing with heart attacks on a daily basis, Dr Audrius Simiatis comments: 'It's uncommon for a heart attack to occur in the female patient before menopause, and very rare for a woman under the age of 40. If you have a female patient younger than 40, it is usually down to either a very unhealthy lifestyle, plus an existing disease (like diabetes), or a significant genetic predisposition.'

Myocardial fibrosis – where 'myo' means muscle and 'cardial' denotes heart – is a condition whereby there's a substantial and abnormal build up of collagen material in the walls of the heart. Fibrosis is essentially a synonym for scarring in the wall of the heart muscle (myocardium). This scarring occurs in the same way as when we cut our skin – we lay down scar tissue to fill the wound. If the cut is deep and substantial enough, the scar becomes a permanent alternative to the skin it's replacing. If the scar is big enough, we often feel a different touch sensation in that area – the scar tissue behaves differently to normal skin. The myocardiocytes (cardiac muscle cells) of the myocardium have a limited ability to repair or regenerate after trauma, so fibrosis can become the heart's permanent work-around post-damage.

Inflammation – we kept hearing this word again and again from all our cardiac experts, especially Dr Parry-Williams. There's an emerging body of thought, to which they all seem to subscribe, that almost all heart disease is actually a synonym for inflammation. All of the heart specialists went out of their way to signpost in bright neon the overarching role inflammation plays in the incidence of heart disease and its manifestation in veteran athletes.

Back to Dr Merghani's study. Both the athlete and control groups then had a cardiac MRI, a process designed to test even the most committed agoraphobic, as it can take an hour and a half wedged into a narrow tube with a tray of equipment across your chest. I'm a fully practising claustrophobic, so my own cardiac MRI for Dr Stephens was made possible only by the sense of humour (when I had all but lost my own) and sensitivity of the superb staff at Paul Strickland Scanner Centre in North London. The objective of the cardiac MRI is to assess whether the structure of the myocardium contains a substrate (a physical layer with alternative specific properties) that's driving arrhythmias.

The result of the athlete and control group cardiac MRI scans made Dr Merghani's research journey even more mysterious. None of the control (sedentary) group, which included males and females, had any myocardial fibrosis at all, and only one female masters athlete showed signs of myocardial fibrosis, but the incidence of one person is not, by nature, of statistical significance and in this instance was considered to be an outlier. To quote Dr Parry-Williams, 'Men veteran athletes get heart abnormalities and women don't.' We will talk a little later on as to why this may be.

However, a 'staggering' (to quote Dr Merghani) 15 per cent of all the male veterans in the athlete group displayed some level of myocardial fibrosis or heart-scarring in the myocardium. Remember, by definition this cohort in this athlete grouping are all super-fit midlife athletes, training at least eight hours a week, and crucially none of them had, so far at least, experienced any adverse symptoms during activity. These are all lifelong exercisers across the spectrum of ability from weekend warriors to world champions. At first glance, this unexpected finding seemed to contain statistical gold dust for the populist exercise-deniers and tabloid press, who inevitably fixated on the fact that precisely none of the people in the control group had any myocardial fibrosis at all, compared to 15 per cent of the male athlete cohort.

However, it has to be considered an unintended consequence of the study that it re-energised the tabloid press. Numbers don't lie, but they don't always tell the entire truth. Activity and sport, it has always been presumed, is supposed to be good for us, and more sport therefore would be better. What was happening to the male heart on a cellular level as it progressed from sedentary through to moderate exerciser, and then finally to heavy exerciser? Was Dr Morris entirely wrong all those years ago or were there more subtle mechanisms at play here?

The location of the myocardial fibrosis in the 15 per cent of male athletes who had them was assumed to be important, so we need to understand a little about the structure of the heart muscle at this point. The myocardium or heart muscle is broken into three strata – the inner layer of the heart muscle wall is called the sub-endocardium, the mid-layer is called the mid-myocardium and the thin outer layer is the epicardium. The three coronary arteries are the heart's own private blood supply and they run from the aorta to attach and perfuse (provide blood) at the inner sub-endocardium level. The coronary arteries only supply blood to the body of the heart muscle itself and are in that sense part of a vital internal circuit.

The Merghani study did identify some myocardial fibrosis at the mid-myocardium and epicardium levels, which was presumed to be caused by inflammation and/or 'myocarditis'. Myocarditis is a new term in our rapidly expanding cardiac lexicon – it is an inflammatory condition that's thought by some doctors to be caused, in athletes at least, by training with a viral infection. This has not been proven beyond doubt and is still contentious, even among cardiologists. Myocarditis is sometimes known as inflammatory cardiomyopathy, but it's worth noting that a small percentage of Dr Merghani's athlete cohort displayed myocardial fibrosis that could have a root cause in myocarditis, inflammation or some other cause that has yet to be established and explained. Dr Stephens offers another plausible explanation: 'The most likely mechanism of fibrosis – which is real, I'm sure – is chronic stretch due to thousands of hours of high cardiac output.'

The majority of the athlete group that showed myocardial fibrosis, however, did so at the sub-endocardium level – which, remember, is perfused by the coronary arteries. If there was a partial narrowing of the space (stenosis) in one of the coronary arteries, it's feasible that under heavy cardiac demands there could be a myocardial ischemia or reduced blood flow to the heart muscle. This could cause part of the heart to be deprived of oxygen and then be remodelled (a euphemism for 'die'). The heart wall cells that die would theoretically, as we know, be filled with scarring material or myocardial fibrosis. And what could possibly cause a partial blockage? The most obvious perpetrator, Dr Merghani's research team hypothecated, would be a coronary artery atherosclerosis, or plaque.

Tracking plaques

All of the Merghani study groups – athlete and control – were subjected to a coronary CT scan, which counts calcium molecules in a defined volume to give a calcium, or Agatston, score. Dr Stephens explained this mechanism in his very distinct way at a recent lecture: 'The inflammatory cells that seem to be at work contributing to the formation of plaques express bone proteins – god knows why – and attract calcium into themselves and lay down calcium.'

When Dr Merghani reviewed the data from the CT scans, there seemed be a clear and concerning trend that implicated only the male athlete cohort. The female athletes, and the male and female control groups (sedentary to moderate exercisers), showed consistently low coronary calcium scores and a low incidence of coronary plaques (lesions). In contrast, the male athlete group had significantly higher coronary calcium scores than the control and female athletes. In addition, substantially more of the male athlete group had atherosclerotic plaques (a build-up in the arteries) than the female athletes and control group, and an even higher percentage had multiple lesions or plaques. In fact, seven per cent of the male athlete group had prevalence of a greater than 50 per cent stenosis (narrowing) of a coronary artery – meaning that a key coronary artery was more than 50% blocked. None of the other groups (i.e. female athlete, female sedentary, male sedentary) had any incidence at all.

These findings were entirely unexpected and somewhat inexplicable – the very thing that was supposed to be protecting us, i.e. exercise, appeared to have the potential to fatally harm those of us males who choose to exercise immoderately. It begged so many supplementary questions about how much exercise is too much, and what steps could be put in place to ameliorate the worst effects of immoderate exercise? Worst of all, it looked like the tabloid articles about too much exercise, especially into middle age, might just be right – always a worrying outcome. Going back a few decades and did Jim Fixx in fact run himself to death, as the exercise-deniers claimed at the time, and could he have lived longer if he had been a more moderate exerciser?

Dr Simiatis posits a possible mechanism for the increased calcium scores and plaque lesions seen in the male veteran athletes: 'The mechanism that's driving the increased CAC (Cornoary Artery Calcium) score, I think, is "shear" strain. During long endurance rides and runs our arteries are exposed to a tenfold increase of blood flow through our arterial system, a 20 per cent increase in diameter, and a sixfold increase in shear stress. Inevitably this will cause micro-trauma to the small structures of the coronary arteries and body, which will repair these micro-injuries through various mechanisms, including the deposition of calcium.'

Atherosclerotic plaques (an unwanted build-up of blockages in the coronary arteries) are a pivotal and fascinating subject, and we'll be returning to their actual composition very soon. Before we do, let's get more of the apparent bad news out of the way. And breathe.

Cardio-toxic: An exercise-dose relationship?

The Merghani team dug down into the data a little further to try to establish some clarity around exercise dosing, in terms of both duration and intensity. They first plotted atherosclerotic calcification (calcium deposits in the artery) against the number of kilometres cycled. This clearly showed a marked decline in coronary calcification as the distance cycled increased from zero through to a deflection point at around 100km per week. At 100km, you can see the curve turns positive as coronary calcification actually increases quite steeply as you cycle into and beyond 150km per week. This J-Curve paradox is also reflected in exercise intensity with a similar deflection based on how hard the training sessions are. This is a harder metric to track because at least some of the data is based on the individual's perception of effort. The specific conclusion of the Merghani research appears to be that cycling is positive up to around 100km as the calcium deposits decline as the distance ridden increases. But then the curve changes shape and the calcium deposits increase with the kilometres ridden over 100km per week.

It is worth restating that all the way to the 100km per week distance, there's no debate at all that all the changes are hugely positive – the risk of obesity, high blood pressure, AF (atrial fibrillation) and CHD (coronary heart disease) are all substantially reduced. There's also a 13–20 per cent decrease in cardiac mortality per metabolic equivalent of task (MET). MET is a scale to measure your exercise rate relative to your baseline resting rate.

A huge US study of 44,452 males over 12 years from 1986 to 1998 concluded a wholly and inverse relationship between activity levels (such as running, weight training and walking) and CHD. The men who ran up to an hour a week had an almost 50 per cent drop in CHD risk over their sedentary colleagues. What seems to be unambiguous from all the studies is that the benefits of exercise are huge and beyond the efficacy of any drug ever invented. Moreover, the benefits of activity are tremendously front-loaded in terms of intensity and duration, which is fantastic news and motivation for the sedentary individual who seeks to become more active, but right now speaks no wisdom to middle-aged men who enjoy being immoderate.

Speaking of which, it's time for some more bad news (on the surface, at least). I would say that the Merghani J-Curve can be seen as somewhat allegorical for the whole of this part of the book. There's a rebound coming, I promise, where we dispel some of the myths and hold some of the worst prophecies and conclusions up to the light. It's my decision alone to front-load all the anxiety and fear in this chapter, partly because I think you can take it and partly because we all like a rebound.

The troponin story

At first glance the troponin story doesn't necessarily make good bedtime reading if you're a midlife cyclist. Troponins are a group of proteins found in both skeletal and cardiac muscle – their role is to regulate contractions of both. Troponin leaks out of the cells of the myocardium (heart muscle) during a heart attack and as a consequence will be counted when the person is being treated, either by a first responder or at the hospital. Somewhat unhelpfully, the troponin levels of heart attack victims and endurance athletes post-event can be very similar. Just when we didn't need another paradox.

A recent study followed 28 runners through the 2017 Brighton Marathon. Their cardiac troponin (cTn) was measured pre- and post-event. Straight after the event and for the following three hours, the study found troponin levels for all participants exceeded the threshold for myocardial infarction (heart attack).

But the mechanisms at play for exercise-induced elevated troponin levels seem to be different from those involved in a heart attack – not least because of the speed of decline in cTn levels. In the marathon-runner group their troponin levels rapidly dropped in the intervening 24 hours post-event; in contrast troponin levels in heart attack patients can stay elevated for a week, suggesting different biological mechanisms are at work. This led the Brighton study of Baker, Leckie, Harrington and Richardson to conclude: 'In the short term, these (28) individuals show no increased risk of cardiac events; however long-term data is lacking.'

Right now, the troponin story is a whodunnit in progress – a euphemism for 'we don't really know'. We will have a load more unknowns before this chapter is out. But possibly none at all when this book is revised in 20 years' time. It is perfectly possible that raised troponin levels are an entirely benign, possibly even defensive, response of the body to a huge slug of rigorous exercise, one of the body's ways of adapting to high-level training. We simply don't know if raised athlete troponin levels are a cause or effect. And do they in fact presage fibrosis? The clue lies in the quote above ('long-term data is lacking'), but we still have to make the best decisions we can as responsible adults while scientific history is being written. Dr Stephens comments from the front line, dealing with midlife athletes every day: 'The key is the very early rise and rapid fall in troponin. Completely different kinetics to MI (myocardial infarction or heart attack). It's seen in all marathoners. No collateral evidence of damage. Many think it [troponin] is functioning as a signal molecule in this situation. The main issue is erroneous diagnosis in collapse after challenge-type events.'

The main issue Dr Stephens is highlighting is when midlife athletes are misdiagnosed, post-event, as having had a cardiac event when elevated troponin is common to all participants. One hopes this is less of an issue now as more research on elevated troponin levels is published.

It's a set of symptoms that our other treating cardiologist, Dr Simiatis, is also very aware of: 'I was thinking more about troponins. For example, in hypertension, when increased blood pressure results in an oxygen supply-demand mismatch, we observe a troponin rise. It does not mean that a patient had heart attack, it is just a reflection of myocytes (muscle cell) breakdown. With vigorous exercise for a prolonged time, athletes definitely have a oxygen supply-demand mismatch and as a result of this, troponin leak will be inevitable. We know for sure that skeletal muscle breakdown occurs after vigorous exercise and is widely accepted as an adaptation mechanism, which is beneficial long term. So why are we concerned about small troponin leaks after vigorous exercise? The only possible exception here might be that if a troponin leak exceeded a certain threshold which is yet to be established by future studies, this might indicate pre-existing coronary artery or heart muscle disease.'

Both of the treating cardiologists, Drs Stephens and Simiatis, both self-confessed immoderate cyclists, take a fairly relaxed view of midlife athlete post-exercise troponin release. It is documented, it happens, but we're yet to see the harm.

Are all plaques equal?

Just so you know, we've now firmly rebounded off the bottom of the bad-news J-Curve. The hypochondriacs among you can now come out from behind the sofa. The rest of this chapter is a presentation of the counter-evidence, or at the very least, a discussion around some of the plausible mitigating circumstances. We've heard from the prosecution and it's now time for the defence.

If you remember, we left the plaque story sounding pretty negative – over 100km per week seemed to be implicated in a notably greater burden of atherosclerotic plaques in our male veteran athlete cohort. It's hard to see a silver lining inside those congested coronary arteries, but there is one if we look carefully enough.

The huge clue is in plaque morphology. Other studies have shown the J-Curve relationship between exercise and atherosclerosis in veteran athletes, but the Merghani group took it one stage further and carefully examined the plaque constructs using a CT coronary angiogram, which shows the blood flow using an injected marker dye in the blood.

As we learned earlier, plaques come in three distinct varieties – soft, calcified and mixed. Soft plaques are just as they sound – fatty and soft and made up almost entirely of malleable lipids (fats) and cholesterol. They are intrinsically unstable and can quickly and easily get inflamed and rupture, which can trigger a clot when the fatty contents of the plaque meet oxygen-rich blood in the artery. This may cause the artery to block completely and a heart attack or myocardial infarction (MI) will ensue. Calcified plaques are quite hard and stable, and while they do have mass and can cause a partial blockage or stenosis, they are inherently less likely to rupture, thrombose (form a blood clot) and block the artery. Mixed plaques are a combination of soft and calcific plaques and are themselves unstable.

Dr Merghani's study appeared to show that the female control group and the female athlete group actually had very similar plaque morphology – their atherosclerotic plaques were mainly calcific in structure. The only difference was that the female athletes had around 10 per cent mixed plaques and the control group had around 10 per cent soft plaques.

However, the male control group had different plaque architecture compared to the male athlete cohort. The male control group (sedentary/moderate exercisers) had on average around 70 per cent soft and mixed plaques, with only 30 per cent of their plaques being calcified in composition. Incidentally, Dr Parry-Williams thinks that inflamed mixed material plaques have the potential to be the most unstable of all – even more than soft plaques.

The male athlete group, however, had mainly calcific plaques (70 per cent). So, even though the male athlete group had a higher burden of atherosclerotic plaques in terms of sheer numbers, it's thought that the individuals were better protected from rupture, clotting and heart attacks because the morphology of their plaques was over 70 per cent calcific. In that sense, exercise is acting like statins (drugs that reduce cholesterol production) by changing the structure of plaques from soft and mixed to calcific. Dr Merghani even speculated to me, while we were talking, that the development of calcific atherosclerosis in veteran athletes may even be a protective process! That's an astonishing thought – the very thing that has fuelled the hysterical media may be an adapted mechanism that's protecting veteran sports people from damage. Add this to the list of unknowns, but I think it's highly significant that a cardiologist like Dr Merghani would even float this out for debate. It's a breathtaking thought.

Shape-shifting plaques

Statins are now one of the most prescribed drugs to men and women of a certain age. Statins are prescribed because they reduce low-density lipoprotein (LDL) – often nicknamed 'bad cholesterol' – which distributes fat molecules around our bodies. Cholesterol has an intrinisic role in preserving nerve function and also for cell wall production. Statins actually work by impeding an enzyme called HMG-CoA-Reductase. The pharmaceutical name for statins is HMG-CoA reductase inhibitors. Enzymes are biological firelighters – they initiate and speed up vital biological processes. In this particular instance – the formation of LDL cholesterol – it is thought that statins act like high-intensity exercise and make the plaques more calcific and therefore stable.

LDL struggles to get good reviews in the mainstream media and has become the pantomime villain of cardiovascular disease – a heart-throb for all the wrong reasons. LDL is actually an essential part of a mechanism that transports lipid (fat) molecules around our bodies to be used by our cells. It's thought that excessive oxidisation of LDL within the coronary arteries can lead to adverse plaque build-up.

In contrast, high-density lipoprotein (HDL) is thought to have a wholly benevolent influence on our constitutions. HDL is a composite of a number of proteins – its role is to export excess cholesterol and triglycerides (a compound made up of three fatty acids and glycerol or glucose) away from cells that have a surplus of both. HDL is often referred to by doctors as 'good cholesterol', on the assumption that a good HDL/LDL balance will regulate the formation of soft and mixed plaques in our coronary arteries.

Midlife cyclists who have been cycling for many years may have more atherosclerotic plaques than sedentary people of the same age, but Dr Stephens thinks this may be a red herring, in the sense that high-level exercise seems to have a mechanism similar to the action of statins, by removing softer, more troublesome material from the coronary artery wall. This is strongly redolent of the earlier observation from O'Keefe et al.: 'Physical exercise, though not a drug, possesses many traits of a powerful pharmacological agent.'

Exercise is, it seems, nature's very own statin and can have the same dynamic effects on plaque morphology. But it should also be clear that born-again athletes, and those coming to intense cycling or running after a largely sedentary life, may be facing a differing risk profile when it comes to plaque morphology. All the cardiologists we spoke to overwhelmingly endorsed and supported taking up exercise in midlife and beyond (especially Drs Stephens and Simiatis), but the exercise dosing and clinical support may be subtly different.

So where are the bodies?

The question of where the bodies are came out of a note sent to me by Dr Stephens. I'm not sure if it originated with Dr Stephens, but it certainly fits his wonderfully dry take on clinical matters. He (appropriately) always seems to find his way to the very heart of the matter. His point is well taken – if high-level cycling into middle age is dangerous, why are we not dying in big numbers?

Some of what has emerged in this section of the book can be interpreted as worrying, alarming even. Dr Stephens' comment was intended to calmly anchor us all in common sense, encourage us to look at the empirical evidence and not to get hysterical or become part of the worried well.

The emerging research on veteran athlete health seems to coalesce around several themes, which are worth summarising. Firstly, there does seem to be an increased prevalence of heart muscle scarring (mycocardial fibrosis) associated with high doses of veteran cycling and running. Dr Merghani's study found a statistically significant 15 per cent uplift compared to the control group, which had zero per cent. The fibrosis could itself be causing arrythmias as the damaged heart tissue interferes with the heart's internal circuitry. Dr Merghani also accepts that there are unanswered questions around the incidence of veteran sportsman fibrosis and suggested to us in an interview: 'The cause for the fibrosis is not certain – there were different patterns of fibrosis and these patterns are associated with different causes.' Presumably, therefore, there must be other factors: one is demand ischaemia – during maximum stress effort, the coronary circulation is temporarily unable to meet the demand of the heart muscle. The other is inflammation – that mysterious word again! We discuss this at length in the final chapter, 'The Mindful Cyclist'.

It's possible that protracted, hard endurance efforts can result in myocardial fibrosis in some high-mileage veteran male cyclists and runners. That would normally be a cause for concern in sedentary individuals of the same age, but we don't know if the fibrosis is leading to damaging arrythmias until the results of longitudinal studies are analysed. Going back to Dr Stephens' question about the lack of bodies – 1:50,000 in the London Marathon, and 1:36,000 in Ride London are clearly very low death rates for a heart issue that's assumed to be prevalent in a huge number of us. It's also worth restating that both the London Marathon and Ride London are overwhelmingly well-represented by veteran male athletes between the ages of 40 and 70. One of the founding fathers of the subject of sports cardiac health and athletic participation was Dr Dan Tunstall Pedoe, the original Chief Medical Officer for the London Marathon, a post he held for 27 years. Dr Tunstall Pedoe assiduously kept records of all the medical incidents during his time in the post. When questioned about the very low rates of sudden death in the event he was apparently heard to remark (one presumes, only half-jokingly): 'Maybe if they were going to die, they died in training.'

I put this point to Dr Parry-Williams who, while appreciating Dan's deadpan humour, disagreed with the medical conclusion. Her own view is that on event day there are hypothetically many more additional elements that could potentially lead to a cardiac incident than in training. Again none of this is proven and has to be added to our 'unknown' cardiac in-tray, but Dr Parry-Williams suggests that our inflammation burden on our event days could actually be markedly higher than in training due to factors such as lack of sleep, nerves, adrenaline, too much caffeine, dehydration or hyponatremia (low sodium due to too much water), event-day effort levels that haven't been adequately trained for, too many high-sugar supplements and snacks, and so on. We'll return in more detail to inflammation and its possible mitigation, but one of our experts thought that we're probably more likely to have a cardiac incident in an event than in training. And the fact that the evidence shows that we do not suggests that there's a mechanism of adapted protection in our hearts which counters the possible increased fibrosis.

The second theme, and the most media-agitated, is the atherosclerosis story – the increased incidence of plaques in veteran male athletes. This is the one that the tabloids have run and run with because atherosclerosis is an assumed close cousin to myocardial infarction (heart attack) and death. And I think this returns us to one of the cornerstones of this book – that there has never been a genetic imperative in keeping humans, but especially men, alive beyond their 20s, never mind their 50s! Training and racing hard into middle age is a highly personal choice and, to some degree at least, an experiment.

The very early stages of coronary atherosclerosis were in fact found in young men who died in the Korean War in the 1950s. The Armed Forces Institute of Pathology in the USA found that 77 per cent of young soldiers had early-stage atherosclerosis upon autopsy – many of these men were under 20 years old. Atherosclerosis is in that sense something that men live with – its antecedents are always in us from a very early age. Dr Simiatis has a pragmatic approach: 'Atherosclerosis constitutes a challenge for the entire cardiovascular community. We doctors have identified the process of atherosclerosis in fine detail [and] invented multiple medications to prolong survival from various cardiac conditions. We can abort heart attacks using highly sophisticated equipment and keyhole surgery that deploys stents through a 2mm (0.08in) hole in the wrist. If the patient gets in touch promptly after the onset of heart-attack symptoms, they can potentially be discharged 48 hours after admission, suffering minimal consequences. Doctors can also conduct open-heart surgery with superb long-term results and implant high-tech pacemakers the size of half a matchbox that can deal not only with electrical heart conduction problems, but with heart failure. And failing all else, we can even transplant a new heart! Despite this, are we ever going to completely beat atherosclerosis? Once we're born, abandoning this earthly world is inevitable. Maybe the very early stages of atherosclerosis as witnessed in the foetus is an enshrined mechanism to leave this world at some later stage.

Drs Simiatis and Stephens may well be right – that atherosclerosis is an intrinsic part of the majority of men's DNA and is present relatively early in life for them. The propensity for atherosclerosis has never been genetically selected out, because until very recently we would be dead long before its worst effects could harm us. We would have died in battle, cut ourselves and died of an infection, or succumbed to a whole host of diseases that prevented us getting anywhere near what we now refer to as middle age. And yet in terms of veteran athlete health, atherosclerosis is something of a red herring. Moreover, it appears that midlife athletes could be better safeguarded than the inactive population precisely because of the protective effect of the morphology of their plaques. Dr Merghani even suggested that there may even be a protective effect of calcification. Dr Simiatis wonders whether declining collagen contributes to our increased incidence of atherosclerosis and proposes a new clinical trial involving the administering of collagen supplements to midlife athletes: 'Collagen is everywhere in the body, including in the wall of coronary arteries. As the result of this, coronary arteries lose their elasticity and become much less resistant to shear stress. We know that once we are over the age of 25, every year we lose one per cent of our collagen, which means that by the time we're 55 we've lost 30 per cent of our collagen.'

The third recurrent cardiac theme is veteran athlete arrythmias. The link between fibrosis and arrythmias may not be fully understood, but nobody currently doubts the existence of a four- or fivefold frequency of atrial arrythmias in the male veteran athlete population, compared to those who are sedentary. Atrial arrythmias in older sports people were first described by Dr Stephens and Professor Greg Whyte, when they started to see disproportionally higher numbers of middle-aged athletes with abnormal heart rhythms than they would expect to see in that age group.

Atrial arrythmias are thought to be caused by the atria (the top chambers of the heart) of older sports people (mostly men) losing elasticity over time because of decades of exposure to prolonged and intense exercise. The atrial stretch is assumed to the underlying driver in abnormal heart rhythms in older endurance sports participants as the atria lose their elasticity and become permanently enlarged. Dr Stephens says: 'Atrial arrythmias are real and they are also the most common "proper" cardiology concern I see in masters sportsmen.'

Dr Merghani speculates about the far higher prevalence of atrial arrythmias in men compared to women: 'Atrial arrhythmias are more common in men. No one knows the exact reason, but a popular theory is that oestrogen [in women] allows the heart to be more compliant and less prone to stretch and scarring.'

The title of this chapter is 'Will I Die?' and, although atrial arrythmias are fairly common in lifelong, endurance-based, male heavy exercisers, they are very treatable and are unlikely to kill you, or even necessarily curtail your cycling activity. Dr Stephens again: 'Atrial arrythmias aren't something where I would want to forbid sport in someone where this is identified.'

I have many clients who have experienced atrial arrythmias. A typical presentation they relate is that they suddenly feel weak and tired on the bike, to the point where it's very hard for them to even turn the pedals over. At the same time, their heart rate monitor shows a significant jump to a very high number, sometimes frighteningly high, beyond even their previously reported maximum. Alternatively, their heart rate begins to fluctuate wildly. The loss of power is common to both circumstances, and they are inevitably compelled to stop cycling, or ride home very slowly. The treatment for atrial arrythmias could be a combination of anti-arrhythmic and anti-coagulant drugs, or a 'catheter ablation' procedure. An ablation involves tiny wires being inserted into a vein in the heart, with the purpose of nullifying the affected heart tissue that's specifically involved with generating the abnormal heart rhythms. The neutralising of the specific part of the heart tissue is achieved using high-frequency radio waves that generate heat. The clients who I know have had ablations are all riding now symptom-free. (see case study I, p. 266). Consequently, atrial arrhythmias are indeed relatively common but they are also well understood, very treatable and for the purposes of this section of the book, very unlikely to kill us.

'No purity in medicine'

This quote is attributable to Dr Parry-Williams, and every one of our four contributing experts went out of their way to rise above the research and data to make a crucial point that athletes tend to live longer, in greater physical and mental health, than inactive folk. Lifelong athletes (those who have been constantly exercising hard for 20 or 30 years) seem to have subtly remodelled hearts that somewhat break normal rules. It's finally being observed and recognised that veteran high-dose exercisers don't necessarily follow the established pathologies of their sedentary contemporaries. The athletic heart seems to be different. A finding of fibrosis, arrythmias and atherosclerotic plaques in a 50-year-old non-athlete would almost certainly raise medical eyebrows and probably trigger all kinds of medical interventions. But in a masters sportsman, the reaction may be much more circumspect, specifically because we seem to be a distinct category to the moderate exerciser or sedentary population.

Remember the 52-year-old cyclist in Dr Merghani's study, who had a 14-beat run of ventricular tachycardia (VT)? (See page 77.) This would normally be so much of a concern that some cardiologists would quickly fit an implantable cardioverter defibrillator (ICD), which would shock the individual if he went from VT into a potentially fatal ventricular flutter (VF). Well, this individual is still alive and well and still training hard and presumably still has occasional 14-beat runs of VT. Furthermore, all the veteran athletes who participated in the study are still alive and doubtless still subjecting themselves to high-intensity and high-duration training doses.

There is, however, no disguising the fact that there are still many baffling unknowns around long-term heavy exercise and (mostly male) midlife athletes:

- What are the drivers of male veteran athlete fibrosis?
- Does fibrosis link to arrhythmias in veteran athletes?
- What role does elevated troponin play in the veteran heart story, if any?
- What process is driving increased atherosclerosis in men?
- What mechanism is at work in creating veteran athlete arrythmias and is there anything we can do to ameliorate them?
- Why are male veteran athletes generally more exposed to cardiac risk than female veteran athletes?
- Does oestrogen provide a protective effect for the female athlete (pre-menopause)?
- Is testosterone a contributor to the increased male cardiac risk associated with high-dose exercise?
- What role does inflammation play in masters athlete cardiac risk and health?

So what now? We have a huge pile of known unknowns, and a vaguely worrying pile of empirically observed issues, which seem to correlate in multiple studies to selective cardiac restructuring, in response to the high-dose exercising of midlife cyclists. On the other hand, the vast majority of us seem to be resilient, healthy and high-functioning on our high-dose exercise diets, and we're cognitively protected, too. But is the heart remodelling adaptive and desirable, or auguring future problems?

Both our cycling cardiologists take a wonderfully pragmatic view of their own immoderate approach to their respective cycling careers. Dr Stephens is seeking to become world champion in his age category on the track, and is very clear about his own personal risk/reward algorithm: 'I train and race bicycles at this level because I enjoy it, not because I think it is necessarily good for me.'

Dr Simiatis mirrors this sentiment. When I ask him to question his own risk/reward strategy when it comes to cycling, he says: 'Once I'm on the bike in the Alps conquering various cols or fighting with L'Étape timelines, I'm 100 per cent cyclist, there's no trace of cardiologist in my mind.'

I adore these reflections from these two specialists. In a way, they sum up so much of this book. Many of us cycle hard into and beyond middle age just because we can, to celebrate the opportunity to elongate a high-performance lifestyle where our parents and grandparents couldn't or didn't. We cycle hard because it makes us feel good and keeps us mentally sharp. In essence this book seeks to tease out notions of 'could' from 'should' in the face of undeniable genetic irrelevance. We certainly can perform at an alarmingly high level on our bikes. Dr Stephens can sustain 50km/h on the track and on the road. In fact, I have many clients who are chasing power outputs of five watts per kilogram of body weight well into their 50s! I'm inspired and astonished by what my clients and friends achieve on their bikes every day. Nevertheless, that does still leave the question of whether we *should* pursue this level of performance into middle age. At least, what else should we do to protect ourselves as best we can in the face of so many unknowns?

Mitigating the risk

One more time for the record: taken in the round, physical exercise has a miraculous effect, both on our longevity and the quality of our lives. But for a small number of people, protracted high-intensity exercise into middle age carries a risk. This is the prevailing wisdom inside the research teams of Drs Ahmed Merghani and Gemma Parry-Williams. Everything they do is attempting to identify these individuals, so they can be better informed and protected, and at the same time establish empirically verifiable trends around exercise dosing in the more mature athlete, which will help all of us. Hence current gold standard strategies around managing cardiac risk associated with high-dosing exercise into middle age can be divided into approaches that are probably relevant to all of us, and others that are specific to differing groups based on sex, medical history and athletic record.

The sex divergence around midlife athlete cardiac risk has only been recently documented and does seem to reveal a rather startling state of affairs. Professor Sanjay Sharma – chief medic to the London Marathon and one of the country's most senior cardiac academics – expresses it this way about a recent study: 'Females were rather boring, in the nicest possible way. They showed nothing – no atrial fibrillation (AF), no scarring (fibrosis), no calcification in their arteries. The day you show me a veteran female athlete who has increased atherosclerosis (coronary artery plaques), I will believe that too much exercise is bad for you. Until then I don't believe it!'

So this is one of the rare occasions in life that it's good to be boring. But why is it that many masters women train and race as hard as veteran men, and yet seem to be entirely protected from fibrosis, arrythmias and arthrosclerosis? Why is that and will it change post-menopause when oestrogen levels decline? There's a popular theory that oestrogen may facilitate the heart muscle being more elastic and therefore less prone to stretching and scarring. Conversely, is there something about testosterone that actively encourages fibrosis? These are hypotheticals at the moment and therefore get added to the pile of unknowns.

Dr Parry-Williams wonders if there are differences in the way that men and women train and manage their athletic lives. Do men tend to train and race with a bit more ego than women, which makes men stray too far into the red zone for too long? Or is this too simplistic, sexist even? Cycling Team Doctor Dr Hulse picks up this theme: 'It's infuriatingly multifactorial! But oestrogen is potentially a big factor. I'd say that, at Ride London or sportive level, the strong women riders will be well-trained and the rest will be much less likely to push themselves. Probably a more "healthy" approach to it. All in complete contrast to many of the males! As the saying goes: "Beware of the ones who think they are fast."'

I was chatting to a friend of mine, Dr Justin Mandeville, about this cardiac sex difference. Dr Mandeville (aged 45) is a superb runner, cyclist, swimmer and triathlete, and also happens to be an NHS intensive care consultant. He went on to describe a recent high-intensity indoor cycling training session, which comprised roughly the same number of male and female participants. The session screamed to a climax, as these things always seem to, at which point four of the male participants (including Dr Mandeville) found themselves in various states of physical distress, resulting in more than one of them actually vomiting as a result of the exertion! Apparently, all the high-level female athletes looked on, appalled and incredulous. Now despite Justin being a trained medical professional and superb athlete, this is hardly a scientific study. But it is a powerful anecdote, whose importance struck Dr Mandeville at the time (presumably as he was bent double, spitting bile). What is it that drove a small group of intelligent, well-trained men to push themselves to physical illness in a small room on a bike that was going absolutely nowhere? Justin freely confessed that he was in considerable distress himself for a while and took a good few moments to recover. I asked Dr Mandeville if he thought that training like this was essentially 'good for him'. His answer was swift and emphatic: 'Of course not!' Which begs the question, why do we do it? What if Dr Parry-Williams' hypothesis is correct and there's also something in male behaviour, as well as in the male genome, that predisposes men to cardiac disease? Does that mean men are likely to put themselves at risk in a whole raft of ways? For example, are we also more likely to train through a virus? And therefore is the incidence of mid-myocardial and epicardial issues (outer levels of the heart muscle) observed by Dr Merghani in male veteran athletes instigated by men's increased propensity to keep riding and running when we have a virus, which may lead to myocarditis (inflammatory cardiomyopathy)?

It's common sense that we shouldn't train through a deleterious virus, but is it mainly men who don't heed this received wisdom? Or is there something about the research studies that self-selects a certain person onto the study and excludes other groups? That is to say, if you are a midlife women athlete who does train to the very outside of the performance/duration envelope *and* will instinctively try to exercise hard through a viral infection, does that possibly mean that you're also less likely to volunteer for a clinical study associated with veteran athlete cardiac health? Or do research studies generally tend to naturally attract the worried well rather than the unworried unwell, Jim Fixxes of this world?

Professor Sharma has come up with a simple but powerful guideline to help us judge whether we should exercise or not. He recommends that if the symptoms are above the neck you could exercise sensibly, but anything below – meaning the chest – means you should rest. Dr Stephens makes the point that, leaving aside the risk for a moment, the actual training effect of exercising with a cold, flu or unspecified virus is highly questionable. It seems there's no value in midlife athletes exercising through any kind of virus or post-viral infection. We don't currently know if training through a virus causes fibrosis in veteran athletes in their mid-myocardial or epicardial levels. But the fact that there's a question mark should be enough to dissuade us from going anywhere near a bike or a pair of running shoes! Remember also Dr Stephens' point that he suspects the training effect of the session will be negligible and that the only consequences are likely to be negative, prolonging the day when you can return to full health and train constructively.

Other than the advice not to train through a virus, all the other evidence points to the fact that female veteran athletes are exposed to little or no risk as a result of high-level training and competition, possibly because they are more successful at managing their exercise-health-life balance. To the point where, in the nicest sense possible, women are of little interest to research cardiologists. Though this does assume that these athletes don't have a family history of heart disease and/or high blood pressure, in which case you may want to see your GP and get a QRISK score. QRISK is a minimally invasive prediction algorithm used by clinicians to determine the likelihood of you having a cardiac event in the next 10 years, expressed in percentage terms. The variables and elements accounted for by the QRISK change over time but usually include age, body mass index (BMI), cholesterol levels, family history, blood pressure, and smoking.

Lifelong male veteran athletes

So what is the best advice for a male, lifelong, heavy exerciser? To recap, lifelong heavy exercise means training for more than eight hours per week for 20–30 years with no significant periods of inactivity. Should you go and get screened, scanned, prodded and poked for signs of heart disease? Screening is a controversial subject because it can be expensive and invasive, as well as carrying risks; it also often throws up unintended findings and consequences, which themselves have dilemmas.

As a lifelong heavy exerciser your cardiovascular system will almost certainly be very different to that of a sedentary person of a similar age. You'll have a slower pulse, a higher VO_2 capacity and quite probably a subtly remodelled heart due to repeated physical efforts over the years. Dr Derek Harrington (one of the consultants behind the Brighton Marathon troponin study and himself a midlife cyclist) shared his views with me: 'No, I don't think we should be routinely screening 50-year-old athletes. The commonest pathology by far will be CHD, most will actually have a normal ECG and a normal ECG certainly does not exclude CHD. Certain high-risk groups should be screened, such as those with a known family history of an inherited cardiac condition. There's no evidence that I'm aware of that screening the general population improves outcomes and the risks of SCD (sudden coronary death) in endurance cycling events seem low.' Dr Stephens takes a similarly pragmatic approach and 'doesn't generally go looking for trouble in lifelong exercisers, and is generally symptom driven.'

Let's explain a little more what Dr Stephens means by the term 'symptom driven':

- Blacking out or fainting during exercise
- Exercised-induced angina or chest pain when exercising
- Training loads remaining the same but performance levels dropping off (though this could be attributed to many other causes, such as viruses, fatigue and overtraining)
- Incidence of obvious AF or arrythmias

Therefore, if you're a male lifelong midlife athlete you would probably be well advised to contemplate the following as a responsible minimum:

- Review your family history of heart disease.
- Make sure you get your cholesterol regularly tested and know your HDL/LDL levels.

- Get your blood pressure checked regularly – all the cardiologists flagged this up as strongly indicative of risk.
- Get your GP or cardiologist to do a QRISK score – this will require a cholesterol score, blood-pressure reading and a review of family history.
- Don't ignore symptoms – see Dr Hulse's case study (see p. 268)

Whether you embark upon more invasive diagnostic tests will depend upon your own situation and psychology. Every cardiologist we spoke to thought exercise was generally highly positive and protective. High-intensity and endurance exercise is, however, a risk to a relatively small number of people, who have clinical predispositions. It's up to you to find your own comfort level here. Personally, I took the view that I was fine and kept on doing what I wanted until I felt symptoms. Even then I (stupidly) ignored the symptoms until the arrythmias were an almost constant distraction. It was only at that point that I sought help; initially from my excellent GP (another cyclist called Dr James Kennedy) and then with Dr Stephens. I'll say in mitigation, that other than the arrythmias I felt completely fine and normal and they went away when I was riding the bike.

As an aside, it's assumed that us lifelong exercisers do know our bodies exceptionally well. We monitor function and performance on an almost daily basis: if one day we cannot climb a hill we normally find comparatively easy, we'll assume fatigue or impending trivial illness and stop riding for a while. We have decades of experience about our own health and performance, and that's invaluable and should never be underestimated. We're both physically protected from the stresses of high-intensity exercise and psychologically shielded – we know how our bodies should feel when they are functioning well and conversely when they aren't. Had I felt weak on my bike *and* had arrythmias, I like to think I would have sought professional help sooner.

New and returning midlife cyclists

It's incontestably a good thing to take up exercise at any time of your life and it is becoming clearer all the time that the health and especially cognitive benefits are close to miraculous. Dr Derek Harrington (of the troponin study, see p. 85) says: 'At my level (and I suspect that includes most of the 40–60 cyclists) I think we are doing far more good than any potential harm. Yes, you may see more AF, but I think more likely we are protecting against CHD (coronary heart disease) rather than increasing risks. Long-term exercise lifelong is best but [there is] still some evidence that exercise in later life is beneficial.'

I'm constantly inspired by clients who arrive for a Cyclefit consultation with the goal of L'Étape du Tour or La Marmotte. Twenty years ago, I was slightly incredulous, but now I know better. These clients will do the hard training and achieve their goals, and they will then set new goals and achieve those as well. They are a new generation of cyclists who rapidly become addicted to the cycling and the sense of freedom and personal challenge it brings. Often these clients are either returning to cycling or new to cycling and many have been sedentary for years or decades. I know very well from the goals they come with that they are looking to be immoderate in their exercise dosing. They are the midlife cyclists. The advice to new or returning athletes who seek to be immoderate in their training and event exercise dosing is slightly different to continuous, lifelong exercisers. To describe them, Dr Stephens uses the term 'exercise naïve'. This is in no way intended in a negative or disparaging way, but signals that their bodies have been in a relatively 'silent' state exercise-wise for years, meaning that they are themselves unaware of possible problems. In addition, he makes it clear that these individuals won't have enjoyed the preventative healthy benefits of exercise experienced by lifelong exercisers. The ever-pragmatic Dr Stephens adapts his screening recommendations for the exercise naïve, precisely to address the unknowns. For those veteran athletes who are returning to training or who are new to strenuous endurance sport, Dr Stephens recommends an exploration of symptoms, as per lifelong exercisers, such as fainting, chest pain and changes in performance, as well as a full QRISK evaluation to assess genetic, clinical and lifestyle issues. Dr Stephens also pre-emptively adds in a coronary artery calcium (CAC) score by way of a cardiac CT scan, for any of those individuals who score intermediate or higher on the QRISK survey. For those athletes who do progress to the CAC score, Dr Stephens establishes the morphology of any atherosclerotic plaques that are found. As we now know, soft fatty plaques and mixed morphology plaques are thought to be more of a hazard than calcific plaques. Based on the results of QRISK and CAC scores, the individual may then progress to other tests. Having been through most of the heart-screening processes myself, I can say it's a highly unpleasant experience, but since we all spend much of our time training with our heart rates in orbit, it can only be educational, and hopefully reassuring, to find out what's happening to our hearts when we push ourselves to the brink of exercise intensity.

We talk more about training and nutrition as a new or returning midlife cyclist later, but purely in terms of heart health I recommend initially avoiding extended periods with your heart at its maximum redline too early in your cycling career. Think about gaining a broader fitness base by letting the road and topography dictate your efforts – harder on the hills and easier on the flats. Avoid sitting on a stationary trainer or indoor cycle with your heart at its maximum in pursuit of the fast lane to an elevated FTP (a person's ability to sustain their highest power reading over a set time – 20 minutes, 1 hour, etc). All-round cycling fitness is about much more than FTP – it's not the only metric in town. Let your body adapt organically and naturally to the new stresses that you're placing it under. Let me emphasise that this is my personal opinion.

This is the screening recommended for a returning or new midlife cyclist:

- Tell your GP what you're planning and let them lead the screening process.
- Don't ignore your own symptoms – chest pain, arrythmias, fainting when exercising, etc.
- Review your family history of heart disease – parents, grand-parents etc?
- Make sure you get your cholesterol regularly tested and know your HDL/LDL levels.
- Get your blood pressure checked regularly – all the cardiologists flagged this up as strongly indicative of risk.
- Get your GP or cardiologist to do a QRISK score – this will require a cholesterol score, a blood pressure reading and a review of family history.
- Move to CAC score and Cardiac CT scan if necessary and directed.
- Consider having a stress/ramp test to see what happens to your heart under load.

The inflammation story

Every one of the cardiologists who contributed to this book flagged inflammation as a major contributor to heart disease of all kinds, although it was also normally the last on the list of potential causes and accompanied by a question mark. The role of inflammation is now being discussed in relation to many serious diseases. As Dr Parry-Williams says: 'There's a fast-growing body of scientific evidence to suggest that inflammation plays a major role in many lifestyle diseases and major killers, including heart disease, dementia, stroke, cancers and even anxiety and depression.'

And do men tend to live their lives in a way that causes a greater inflammation burden than women? Do men drink more coffee, become more dehydrated, eat a poorer diet and consume more alcohol, and are they less able to cope with stress, and more reliant upon or exposed to adrenaline? Is this a component of the gender disparity that we're seeing in the research? All of the elements listed above are known to be inflammatory to varying degrees. But how much they are contributing to the incidence of heart disease is currently unknown and awaiting hard research data.

These questions are compelling for researchers like Dr Parry-Williams, who queries whether excess inflammation may be detrimentally affecting our cardiac health – for example, by lowering our arrhythmia threshold that makes us more susceptible to irregular heart rhythms. Myocarditis is defined as inflammation of the heart muscle and is thought to be responsible for both fibrosis and arrythmias. It seems to be a compelling idea that we should attempt to reduce our inflammation burdens as veteran athletes.

It's worth putting some extra context around the topic of inflammation for veteran athletes, in the sense that it's a double-edged sword. Hard exercise is inherently acutely inflammatory but chronically anti-inflammatory. Sounds contradictory, doesn't it? A physically arduous cycling (or running) event will probably be highly inflammatory right in the moment and even immediately afterwards – possibly related to troponin release. But in the long term, hard physical training is likely to provoke adaptions in the athlete that will chronically (that is, over a time period) bestow a generalised and systemic anti-inflammatory protection for the individual. In that sense, veteran athletes can be said to be beneficially, or 'chronically', protected over time, specifically because of their strenuous efforts. This is an area of special interest to Dr Parry-Williams: 'Athletes spend a huge amount of time in acute sympathetic activation during events, but also a great deal of time with their heart rate coasting along at 40bpm in a parasympathetic phase – this is maybe why athletes tend to live longer.'

Dr Parry-Williams has introduced an emerging and potentially paradigm-shifting topic here – the role of our 'autonomic nervous system' in regulating our systemic equilibrium, and even controlling our general inflammation burden.

The autonomic nervous system (ANS)

To understand Dr Parry-Williams's interest in inflammation and how it may contribute to veteran heart issues, we first need to understand a mysterious facet of our bodily functions called the ANS. While the central nervous system (CNS) deals, among many other things, with our conscious movement and control of the skeletal muscle involved in cycling, walking and running, and so on, the autonomic nervous system (ANS) operates under our awareness radar and is responsible for regulating many of our unconscious functions such as heart rate, cardiac regulation, digestion, rate of respiration, urination, defecation and our pupils' response rate (dilation). Considering the vital nature of its work it's incredible that the ANS is fairly poorly understood by most of us. The ANS itself is divided into further branches, including the yin and yang of the sympathetic nervous system (SNS) and parasympathetic nervous system (PSNS). A person's autonomic tone, at any given point in time, and the attendant avalanche of emotional and chemical changes, is the net result of the constantly changing struggle for control between the SNS and PSNS. How this intricate system ever evolved is truly fantastical – it's an incredibly complex internal check and balance on some of our most vital physical processes.

The sympathetic nervous system (SNS) – fight or flight, the 'yang'

The SNS is ironically named because it's the input that deliberately stresses our system ready for fight or flight. In fact, it's not very 'sympathetic' at all.

When the SNS is in control, our body is in a stress response to any situation that may need us to do battle or run away. As an example, I have a very big golden retriever at home, who although universally friendly, also has a frankly colossal subsonic bark that he hardly ever deploys – unless I'm fast asleep and relaxed in a deep parasympathetic state, and he hears a fox howl outside. At which point he unleashes a Four Horseman of the Apocalypse volley that triggers a lightening sympathetic response in my body – jolts of adrenaline and cortisol (the body's primary stress hormone), a spike in blood pressure, a release of glucose into my bloodstream, and a cranking up of my heart rate and respiration, all in preparation in case I have to fight or flee for my life. Once I have padded back from the kitchen after reassuring him that we are not under a full-frontal fox attack, I am still left with my SNS in dominance. I am wired and I am stressed, and my system is in an inflammatory state. Dr Steve Peters, author of *The Chimp Paradox,* refers to this as my 'chimp state', with the primitive limbic system in superiority. With the 'chimp' in ascendency, the reasoning, gentle and considered 'human' is temporarily subdued, waiting for the danger, where fast dynamic decisions are vital, to be over. The SNS state has evolved to work incredibly quickly so we can deal with threat or danger straight away. All the systems that we need to fight or flee are revved up (muscles, heart, breathing, etc) and all the functions that we don't need in the moment are switched off (such as digestion, urination, etc).

The parasympathetic nervous system (PSNS) – rest, digest, feed and breed, the 'yin'

The parasympathetic nervous system is the 'yin' to the sympathetic nervous system's 'yang'. Both are pulling your vital unconscious functions in opposite directions all the time. The parasympathetic phase is your 'Buddha brain' taking back control and unlocking higher order functions such as rest, recovery, digestion and sexual arousal – being in a PSNS phase allows slower and more contemplative thought. Where the SNS works fast and switches on in the crackle of a synapse to fire up all our flee and fight mechanisms, the decision to decelerate the body into a more introspective and recovery phase is less defined and much more circumspect. This fast snap into SNS and a more circuitous route back to the PSNS phase is hardwired into our neural networks.

We have evolved to be more cautious in the unconscious shift back into the PSNS phase, in case danger still lurks out there. Evidence is emerging that many of us struggle to move effectively back into PSNS and instead stay permanently wired in the fast lane, with our foot to the floor, with the SNS in control. This is almost certainly as a consequence of the type of lives that we now lead, which involve complex, time-limited multitasking allied to ambitious goal-setting. In the ancestral environment, the prompt to move back to PSNS from SNS would be the clear visual and audible cues that danger had passed, which would dial back our cortisol levels to allow our autonomic tone to shift back in favour of a PSNS phase.

The ANS and evolved function

The ANS has quietly been governing some of our most important bodily functions for hundreds of thousands of years. The ANS functions on an antagonistic basis, where either the SNS or PSNS wins overall control based upon the perception of what environment your body is facing at any one time. A dangerous enemy, threat or stress will invoke the rapid blunt power of the SNS; whereas a tranquil time is an opportunity for the body to enter PSNS mode, and the ascendency of resting, restoring, digesting and reflecting. The key word here is 'perception' – our bodies evolved to deal with simpler and more binary times in the ancestral environment, where life was more brutal but also simpler. There was a strict order of needs – security, warmth, nourishment, socialisation and breeding/childcare. The autonomic nervous system's binary switching was perfect for dealing with a dangerous world where the quest for food, shelter and defence of family was paramount. Any doubt at all and the safer evolved default would be the switching into a sympathetic mode to deal with perceived hazards and risk. Those of our ancestors of a genetically more laid-back and hippyish disposition, who defaulted to a parasympathetic state, presumably also died out when the lions they were intensely relaxed about suddenly got hungry and ate them.

To take a 'selfish gene'-centric view, our genes are quite relaxed about how long we live as an organism, provided we live long enough to reproduce. Consequently, the safer strategy is to default enough of the time to being in a stressed SNS mode, so we'll at least avoid danger long enough to procreate. But obviously we no longer live in the ancestral environment, and the risks and challenges we face today are very different. We're essentially using a 250,000-year-old alarm mechanism to stratify risk in a modern environment. No wonder that we're getting highly skewed and inappropriate results. Dr Parry-Williams comments that modern lives are: 'like being in a highly sympathetically activated state when it isn't necessary; that's to say, that there are no conditions necessitating either fight or flight.' (Unlike exercise, where we induce a flight mode by tricking our bodies into thinking we are chasing after or escaping an animal when in fact it's just the other competitor who is on our tail!)

I remember delivering a biomechanics paper to a cycling science conference in 2015 in Munster. The title of the talk was 'Mankind didn't evolve to ride bicycles.' It dealt with the concept that our field of expertise and experience – cycling biomechanics – fundamentally involves the interface between a genome a quarter of a million years old (modern man) and a weird Victorian contraption, whose design was frozen in aspic by inter-war politics. I was excited to be talking at the start of the conference – I believed the talk was a necessary and levelling reappraisal of the subject of cycling performance and biomechanics, before we all inevitably disappeared up our own arses for the next 72 hours. So why, five minutes before I walked on stage, did I suddenly feel stressed, alarmed and tense? Why was my heart beating like I was halfway up Mont Ventoux? Why was adrenaline surging through my veins like I had been drugged? In the audience were friends, peers, medical professionals and academics – there was simply nothing to be alarmed about. I tried to talk to myself as I stood and waited in the wings: 'You daft bugger – what is the worst that can happen here? You shit yourself and all your teeth fall out? Unlikely!' Ironically, I know now that the ability to defecate is actually one of the functions that's switched off when we enter SNS phasing.

There was, of course, nothing to be frightened about, but my 250,000-year-old ANS, specifically my SNS, couldn't assess the risk properly, panicked and threw the lever marked 'danger', which was not helpful when I needed to be calm, cogent and eloquent, not fight a grizzly bear for my lunch.

Do men default more readily to the SNS phase, or do women find it easier to unconsciously, or even consciously, climb back down the SNS phase ladder into a more relaxed and amenable PSNS phase? The mechanism itself is well known – we enter SNS phasing like an express elevator and ease back down to PSNS phasing via a hard-to-navigate rope-ladder. It would be relatively easy to construct a case that men have evolved a slightly differently calibrated autonomic tone bias than women, based on the division of roles in the ancestral environment. Go back 250,000 years and the family group is attacked by marauders or wild animals – everyone will doubtless jolt into a SNS phase, but the individual behaviour response may be different based on gender and a perceived division of roles? Would it be fair to assume that it would be the men's responsibility to be first out of the shelter to wrestle the leopard or attacking neighbour? Would it be the women's job to protect the children from harm? Could it be that men's ANS's have evolved to be more biased towards SNS phasing than women's, and might this further explain a potentially harmful inflammation cascade in the 21st century that's affecting our health?

Even if these suppositions were to be correct, there's still a step missing here – does autonomic tone affect levels of inflammation? A recent paper by Koopman et al. predominantly focussed on the relationship between rheumatoid arthritis, which is a chronic autoimmune inflammatory disease, and ANS function/dysfunction, but they also suggested that 'the ANS may control inflammation in humans.' The paper went on to explore the ANS link to other inflammatory conditions such as systemic lupus, systemic sclerosis and chronic inflammatory bowel disease and said: 'The ANS imbalance could be the result of chronic inflammation, but conversely, it is also possible that changes in the ANS influence inflammation, disease development and severity.'

It appears to be entirely plausible that an individual's chronic (over time) inflammation burden is greater the more time they spend in a SNS phase relative to a parasympathetic phase. I'm of course speculating that men have evolved to spend more time in a SNS phase than women and that creates an inflammation cascade – moreover that nature is, in an evolutionary sense, blindly indifferent to the harm that this may cause us in the process. The first is of course highly speculative.

The snakes and ladders of the ANS

We've learned that the only thing protecting us from an eternally distracting and potentially chronically damaging high heart rate is our parasympathetic nervous system and its ability to talk us down from our stressed sympathetic phase. In 1969, the flight surgeon for the NASA Apollo 11 mission reported that, during the launch phase, the three crew members had the following heart rates:

- Commander Neil Armstrong – 110bpm
- Command Module Pilot Mike Collins – 99bpm
- Lunar Module Pilot Buzz Aldrin – 88bpm

All of their heart rate numbers are astonishing, considering the risk and pressure to which the crew were exposed. In front of the whole world they were attempting something that had a high probability of catastrophic failure, whose corollary was an almost certainly painful, public, and distressing death. One of the most perilous phases of any mission is the launch, when the astronauts sit on thousands of tons of combusting propellent. What is clear is that Buzz Aldrin, as well as being the most effervescent member of the crew, was also the one who was best able to invoke his parasympathetic nervous system, with a heart rate of only 88bpm! Most of the billions of people watching around the globe had much higher heart rates than that – I remember watching enraptured with my dad and I'm pretty sure that both of us were well north of Buzz Aldrin's cardiac tickover. Mike Collins' heart was also loping along at 99bpm, but the withdrawn and taciturn Neil Armstrong, was also the most internally stressed of the crew at 110bpm. I have no idea whether Buzz Aldrin was unconsciously or consciously controlling the switch into a sympathetic phase, but his undoubted success at managing his autonomic tone suggests probably the latter and is an example of phenomenal control of SNS–PSNS balance. By the way, Neil Armstrong's heart rate as he piloted the lunar module to a safe landing space on the moon was 155bpm, which for him was probably close to his aerobic threshold. Armstrong may not have found a way to finely control his PSNS response, but his test pilot training had taught him to function in a highly sympathetic state.

I use the example of heart rate here to illustrate that it may be a little misleading or even simplistic for our more earthly exploration of midlife athletes. As Dr Parry-Williams points out: 'Athletes tend to have "high vagal tone" at rest which explains resting bradycardia and generally low blood pressure at rest.' What Dr Parry-Williams means here is that athletes, and especially immoderate endurance athletes, can flatter to deceive with some of our baseline numbers such as blood pressure and resting pulse because of our enhanced 'vagal tone'. Bradycardia, you may remember from earlier in the chapter, is defined as a low heart rate. Professor Sharma starts to get worried if it's routinely below 35bpm (my resting heart rate was routinely between 32 and 34bpm when I was racing regularly, and may partially explain some of my recent problems – see p.253). The vagus nerve is a cranial nerve that runs from the brain-stem, through the chest area right down into the abdomen. It's a key component of our parasympathetic nervous system, forming a vital information and message flow, back and forth between our brain and our internal organs. The 'tone' aspect refers to its action of persistent parasympathetic forces in response to the sympathetic nervous system in a perpetual tug-of-war, with calm on one side descending into panic on the other.

It appears that athletes enjoy higher levels of vagal tone. Asif Marchaga writes: 'Markers of parasympathetic activity are well known to correlate with exercise capacity with elite athletes exhibiting remarkably high markers of vagal tone'. This gives us yet another unknown – does endurance exercise increase vagal tone or conversely are people with naturally high vagal tone drawn to endurance exercise? Asif Machhada again: 'Now it is very much a chicken and egg story: the correlation between the two could suggest that either exercise enhances vagal tone or that there are certain individuals out there that have higher vagal tone, either due to genetic or environmental factors that make them more tolerant of endurance exercise regimes, or it could be a combination of the two.'

This vagal tone–bradycardia–endurance-training cause and effect conundrum was discussed by Dr Stephens at a recent lecture, where his conclusion fell a little more on the genetic predisposition side: 'Conventional wisdom is that when you're fit your pulse slows [but] – I think it may not be that – I think that bradycardia or high vagal tone may just be genetic good luck. You were born with a slow pulse (or at least a propensity to have a slow pulse when you grew up) and a wider pulse range over which your heart can operate, and therefore a greater range of pumped volumes, and therefore you are naturally good at sport.

Dr Stephens made it clear that he was speculating here, but he's also joining the dots based on his own experience dealing with countless patients who were referred to him with bradycardia symptoms. By asking them more detailed questions about their sporting history as younger individuals, Dr Stephens was able to establish that, as well as having a slow pulse, they were previously innately very good at sport.

On the one hand we're presuming that the high doses of intense exercise we undertake will provoke a sympathetic stress response and will be generally inflammatory upon our bodies, certainly in the short term. On the other hand, we envision that participating in endurance sport will reduce our resting heart rate and improve our parasympathetic response capabilities by improving our vagal tone. But it appears that we cannot rely on heart rate alone to indicate whether our sympathetic/parasympathetic autonomic tone is in a healthy balance at any one point in time. Does heart rate variability (HRV) give us the extra detail we need to assess autonomic tone equilibrium?

Heart rate variability (HRV)

Our hearts don't beat like a grandfather clock, where the space between each tick and tock is predictably uniform as each minute passes. In fact, our heart rhythms contain a perpetual beat-to-beat variation. Heart tempo increases fractionally as we breathe in and decreases as we breathe out – the spaces between the beats are constantly shifting. These tiny fluctuations are called respiratory sinus arrhythmias (RSAs) and are measured in milliseconds. These small beat-to-space shifts are widely thought to be an important part of autonomic system regulation and, consequently, are highly desirable. We think of our bodies being healthier and more resilient when they are synchronous and metronomic, but with HRV the opposite is true – broadly speaking, higher variations between our heartbeats result in better mental and physical health and performance outcomes. HRV is a broad indicator of your cardiovascular responsiveness and competence, where a higher score is a demonstration of your body's ability to change rapidly according to a changing physical and emotional landscape. HRV is used in intensive care for assessing the likely recovery from a myocardial infarction (heart attack) and to assess autonomic function associated with neurological disease.

HRV can decline due to many factors, such as ageing, stress, diabetes and overtraining. It's clearly something that as midlife cyclists we need to protect in order to maintain both our health and performance. In a clinical setting, HRV is easily measured using ECG where three graph deflections are measured, collectively known as the QRS Complex. The main 'R' point is the classic peak we recognise in an ECG read-out and represents the actual event of the heart beat. As a consequence, heart rate variability is characterised by the 'R–R interval' or 'RR variability'. ECG is still the clinical gold standard way of tracking the R-R interval or HRV, but there are now many good commercial devices available (WHOOP, Apple, Fitbit, etc) that us midlife athletes can use to review our psychophysiological health in detail so we can make the best day-to-day training and racing decisions.

If we assume for a moment that tracking heart rate variability to affect our stress inflammation burden is a good thing, we also need to know how we can positively adjust our HRV. In the short term it's possible, with practice, to positively shift your autonomic tone towards a parasympathetic primacy state and HRV using simple breathing techniques like breathing in squares – where you breathe in for a count of four, hold for a count of four, breathe out for a count of four and hold for a count of four. Or try deep diaphragmatic breathing routines where you place a hand on your stomach to make sure it's lifting as you breathe in, and then ensure that the out-breath is longer than the in-breath, such as breathing in for a count of four and out for a count of six. This relaxed breathing is a sign to the autonomic nervous system that there's no clear and present danger and you can return to a parasympathetic state, with increased HRV. These are simple techniques and there are hundreds of variations that will have the same effect. Probably the longest-lasting and most profound effect on HRV and the autonomic nervous system would be to practice meditation to reduce overall systemic stress. I do practice diaphragmatic breathing to 'force' myself to relax and promote a more PSNS state at times of tension and anxiety. The autonomic nervous system is the literal neurological junction of our cardiac–respiratory–nervous system, and breathing and mindfulness techniques are a great way to shift our physical and emotional state. I wish I had known this before I delivered my 2015 lecture – a few minutes of private controlled breathing and I could have pulled myself out from the entirely sympathetic state into which I'd got myself!

There has been so much written, especially recently, propagating the notion that there's an inverse, negative relationship between levels of exercise and health risk. Some of the more evangelical pieces in the national press have even suggested that the relationship is binary – for example, exercise beyond seven hours and you definitely *will* increase your risk of cardiovascular problems. This is misleading, dangerous and almost certainly completely wrong.

However, it's true to say that there are still some unknowns about how the body responds to hard and prolonged exercise as we age. Maybe it's been a neglected area of medicine until now because there haven't been enough of us to make it clinically (and maybe financially) interesting from a research perspective. That's no longer the case. Our generation is the first in our entire species history that wants to extract not just fitness and health but real performance from our bodies as we move into middle age and beyond. With the help of the wonderful clinical research being undertaken, by Dr Gemma Parry-Williams, Dr Ahmed Merghani, Professor Sanjay Sharma and many others around the world, our generation can both be the trailblazers for our children and grandchildren when they become midlife athletes, as well as improve our own physical and cognitive performance into our advancing years. Riding our bikes as we get older is almost certainly a great thing – it's a lot of fun, keeps us sharp and helps us enjoy the performance and condition of the average 25-year-old. Clearly we're trying to speed you through all the green lights that we can, while at the same time helping you intelligently navigate, with the most informed evidence and advice, the occasional amber and red lights when they flash, where it may be wiser to exercise caution or even momentarily apply the brakes. Jumping red lights can be just as bad in the metaphorical world as it is in the real one.

4

MIDLIFE PERFORMANCE – TOO LATE FOR SPEED?

Full disclosure: I'm the last person you should listen to when it comes to structured training. Some of you may want your money back at this juncture. Even when I was racing, I was a somewhat chaotic and scrappy trainer. My basic philosophy was to ride my bike enough in the winter for adventure, fun and relaxation, to be able to race myself match fit-ish in the spring. The bike meant as many things to me then as it does now, and the white heat of competition was only one of them. I was also a racing fatalist – you go out and have great days, and you go out and have bad days. And it was possible to burn a lot of anxious calories fruitlessly attempting to join the dots between the two outcomes, but maybe still nothing would change. Needless to say, this chaotic/hippy ethic put me at odds with most of my teammates, who sought to understand more, so that they could control their racing outcomes. I guess my philosophy was generally predicated on – where was the fun in training so much you thought you could predict the outcome of the race? Or training so little that you couldn't take part in the drama of the race? My perfect scenario was to be fit enough to play the game when the flag dropped to take part in the adventure. I asked Dr Jon Baker, who was a coach with team Dimension Data for four years, to critique my old training 'methodology' and I was quite surprised by his analysis: 'Actually, you had a good structure – a "be-in-the-right-ball-park" endurance base in the winter and speed work in the summer – and a good philosophy, but that isn't what most people do. Maybe due to time limitations, a lot of people do too much high-intensity work, all the time, so there's no progression. I think you would do OK with your simple plan.'

Dr Baker is fundamentally right; sometimes I did do OK with that approach. I remember a 120km road race that I took part in many years ago and it started to snow at the halfway mark. Half the field immediately pulled out – who can say why? Snow wasn't part of their race-plan, or they didn't think they had the skills to handle their bikes in the icy conditions, or just a fear of the unknown? It was too early in the season for me to have 'great legs' but I felt sufficiently strong to see how the day went, and a significant psychological bump when 70 riders went down to 30 after a few snowflakes. By the end of the race our bikes were caked in ice and encrusted snow. I think only a dozen or so daft sods finished and I think I came third or fourth in a 'dancing on ice' sprint. The moral, if there is one, is that I was not the third-fittest rider on the start line, I didn't have the third-highest FTP, but I was rested, relaxed, had had a good breakfast, and was available for whatever lay ahead, so it wasn't much of a stretch for me to embrace the chilled chaos. Even 25 years later I remember the fun and surprise and sense of adventure of the race.

Hence my role in this chapter isn't to implore you to cram in one more sweet-spot session, or necessarily raise the roof of your FTP house, but to get your riding and goals into context, with all the combined wisdom that we should have at our age, or, as King Lear's Fool puts it: 'Thou shouldst not have been old till thou hadst been wise.' (Act 1, Scene 5.)

There are plenty of great books out there that will teach you how to train harder, smarter and faster, and how to become pedantic about structuring sessions, and rigid and monastic in the pursuit of aerobic progress. I'm more interested in the context of utilising the bicycle as a means to enhance your health, fitness and love of life.

Is it ever too late to start cycling?

I long ago abandoned any cynicism about what's possible for anyone, at any age, and what they can achieve in cycling. About the time of Lance Armstrong's *It's Not About The Bike* we started to see a new kind of client who had been moved by Lance's story, and it motivated them to jump in and sign up for L'Étape du Tour. L'Étape had traditionally been a huge day out for club-racers and riders, and defiantly not a Sunday fun run for previously sedentary middle-aged folk, who hadn't got out of breath since their last rugby or netball match, 30 years ago. But almost to a man and woman, they trained hard, practised in the mountains, and finished their L'Étape ahead of the dreaded broom wagon. We've already covered this positive side of Armstrong – he single-handedly threw up the shutters of our magnificent sport and invited everyone, including lots of new female riders, to take part. Up until that point cycling was a very male-dominated, slightly secretive sport. But post-Lance we saw many women come into the sport, maybe initially motivated by Lance's cancer survival story, but soon addicted to the adventure, technology and fitness for their own sake. Many of these new riders would come and see us in the autumn, planning to ride L'Étape in the following summer. L'Étape is a reach for a young fit person; we thought, it was probably unreachable for someone who was untrained, middle-aged and possibly overweight. We started to run riding camps to help our new clients with training, nutrition, hydration, cornering, braking and descending advice.

The experience taught us a few sharp lessons. Firstly, that middle-aged women and men can become well-conditioned athletes in just one year, if they do everything broadly correctly. Secondly, that the bicycle is a uniquely credible tool to support this type of intensive athletic campaign, because it's relatively gentle on knees, hips and backs (if it's set up properly). And thirdly, the experience for the individual is a physical and emotional epiphany – they see themselves and their lives through a different lens. We also learned that when you're staring at point zero, the arc of improvement is both steep and flattering, which helps sustain new riders through some of the more challenging aspects of cycling – physical suffering, weather, falls and even punctures. Riders would surf their initial improved performance on a wave of confidence. Who doesn't like going out and getting a personal best on almost every training ride? We also learned how to deal with the psychology of the inevitable performance plateaus that we all reach when we take part in a hard sport like cycling.

The health v performance spectrum

If we take it as a given that, all other things being equal, we would all rather function on a higher physical and mental plane than a lower one, two questions are immediately provoked. Firstly, what is our ultimate aspiration? And secondly, what's the best route for us to achieve our stated goal? I deliberately used the vapid word 'best' for blatantly self-serving reasons, which will become abundantly clear. For example, if your goal at the age of 58 is to become world age-group pursuit champion, like Dr Stephens, you have to countenance the means to achieve the ends. Being number one in the world, even as an age-grouper (especially as an age-grouper in my opinion – all the rubbish riders stopped long ago), requires a huge amount of lifestyle and training commitments, and these will occupy a high proportion of your waking resources. They just will. If on the other end of the spectrum, you cycle as part of a pick-and-mix of exercise, for transport, relaxation and general life enhancement, and your goal is broadly to stay at this level, then different decisions and commitments will inevitably follow. In terms of your physical and cognitive health, as well as the prospect of extending your lifespan, I think Dr Stephens would agree that the latter plan is a safer bet than the former. To reiterate his words from an earlier chapter: 'I race at this level because I enjoy it, not because I think it is good for me.'

Go right back to chapter 3 and Dr Merghani's J-Curve (see p. 84) and it's uncontentious that cycling for an hour or so per day, with varying intensity, is one of the most life-affirming, life-extending things you can possibly do. It's a stronger drug than any pharmaceutical company ever invented for making us happier, healthier, less stressed and clearer thinking. How much training structure, diagnostics and data do you need to enhance performance at this level? Well, I would suggest whatever makes you happy and helps you enjoy your cycling more. If you're cycling six hours a week, mixed between commuting and recreational miles (this is now broadly me, by the way), and a heart rate monitor and power meter augment your experience and help you improve your fitness and speed, then you should absolutely use them as reference tools. I would certainly implore you to buy the best bike, shoes and wheels you can afford and have them professionally fitted to you, to avoid injury or underperformance.

Moving along the spectrum a little – maybe you've now been nudged off your six hours per week equilibrium by a new goal to ride an event such as the L'Étape, or maybe even a multi-day event in the mountains (mission creep in cycling is almost inevitable once you're hooked). Now that the goal is L'Étape, at the very least you have to navigate a couple of major cols ahead of a broom wagon that's waiting to sweep you up and end your day. This new goal will presumably provoke a re-evaluated training plan and methodology consistent with the elevated demands that will be placed on your body. You may think this is the point that you should get yourself checked over by your GP – blood-pressure, ECG, cholesterol, etc. You may even decide that it's rational to employ a coach to set training plans and numbers for you to work to. A ride is no longer a ride for its own sake – it has a stated aim and directive, and therefore a satisfactory or unsatisfactory outcome. How you view this new training structure probably depends upon how you view your entire life. For me, it would feel imprisoning and constraining – that's to say, the price of liberating more power (if it did) would simply be too high in terms of my own personal freedom. I don't want a ride to be preordained or prescribed, I want it to unfold according to my changing mood – feel good, ride fast; feel rubbish, back off and look at nature. But maybe also that's why I was just a good club rider and no more – only good on the right course and on the right day – that was my plateau. I do recognise, by the way, that my Big Lebowski philosophy is unlikely to stand the test if I tried to step up to Dr Stephens' level (now there's a thought for the next book. Can Big Lebowskis ever become world champions?). For other folk, clicking through highly stratified intermediate goals on the way to a longer term principal goal would be both reassuring and satisfying. It depends on how you view other aspects of your life.

The broad principle of training can be reduced to one unassailable statement – human beings are adaptable organisms. Cut yourself, and a scab will miraculously form in a matter of hours and your skin will completely heal in a matter of days. It is a first aid kit that we carry inside ourselves all the time and of course all take for granted, unless of course if it doesn't work. We are not fixed or immutable beings, we're plastic and mouldable – physically and mentally. We can't instantly transform ourselves like superheroes by changing our costume, but we can shift our environment, which in turn will lead to fundamental cellular revision – in the sense that we can expose our bodies to new loads and exertions, which cause them to adapt and change.

Senescence to superhero

We learned in chapter 2 that ageing happens at a cellular level, and that this is called senescence. Our cells lose their ability to copy and divide themselves as accurately as they could when we were younger. But one of the huge advantages of living beyond our evolutionary design life is that we can now exploit mechanisms that are not perhaps as affected by ageing at a cellular level, and one of those is training adaption. In short – we may get old from our cells up, but we also get fit from our cells up. Dr Dave Hulse has a great bedside manner on the subject: 'When we train the aerobic and anaerobic energy systems, what we're training are the biochemical processes that occur within this little structure called the "mitochondria". Crucially, the biochemical systems that provide the energy within the muscle, that then provide force, don't change significantly.'

Maybe this explains why Dr Stephens, at 59, has a virtually identical power output aged 49. He could ride a 16km time trial 10 years ago in just over 20 minutes, and he still can now. That should inspire all of us. Being able to sustain an average speed of almost 50km/h at almost 50 years of age is impressive; being able to sustain that speed at almost 60 years of age is profound. Obviously, his body is still adapting very well to the appropriate kind of training stimulus.

To understand what is happening on a cellular level as we train, we have to do a deep dive into sports science. Dr Hulse again: 'Physical fitness and performance can be defined as the ability of the organism, or parts of the organism, which really means the mitochondria and muscles, to deliver energy and force.'

The mitochondria are tiny, mystical 'organelles' – subcellular entities, which perform a very specific function inside a cell. The crucial role of the mitochondria is that they are the battery pack, or energy source, of our cells – they keep our lights on. Some cells are particularly mitochondria-rich because they have extremely high energy requirements, predictably our brains, hearts and muscles. By delivering the correct training dose or stimulus we can increase the number and size of the mitochondria in our crucial cells, which in turn decreases the distance between the blood flow and the mitochondrial energy source within the muscle itself. There will be a clear and discernible difference in the number and density of mitochondria between a trained and untrained muscle. Our hair and teeth may drop out, we may have creaky backs and can't remember where the car keys are, but our ability to increase our mitochondrial density remains largely undiminished as we move into and beyond middle age – my cup overfloweth. Dr Hulse puts it in team-doctor speak: 'Upregulating the chemical processes themselves, and altering the number and size of mitochondria at a microcellular level, those are the adaptions to training. Whatever we do on a bike, long steady states or intense intervals, we're just trying to effect "subcellular organelle metabolic uplift".'

Quite so! There's also emerging evidence that intense efforts have a proportionally greater net effect on increasing mitochondria density than long, steady-state riding. I was, of course, willing it to be the other way around.

So, we're getting fit from our cells up, but how does that impact our disparate cycling aspirations, and how should we organise our own training if we seek to maximise the stimulus v adaptation effect?

Granularity v barefoot cycling

Thankfully, the thinking around training at all levels is changing. For a while it seemed like you needed a sports science degree to have a hope of getting round a local charity ride for your kid's school. On a subliminal level I'm sure we convinced ourselves that, just as there's a question mark over whether a falling tree actually makes a sound in the woods if nobody is around to hear it, a training ride may not actually happen if it isn't simultaneously recorded and tracked by a power meter and Strava.

The sports industry has, I feel, been guilty of slicing and dicing training levels and data, to the point of unhelpful incomprehension: *threshold, sub-threshold, super-threshold, recovery-aerobic, lactate-threshold, super-aerobic efforts* were all thought to have their place in the professional peloton, which unhelpfully trickled down to us. Did any of this overthinking and overanalysing actually make a single person faster and fitter? It did, of course, sell an awful lot of training programmes, power meters and heart rate monitors. Even the professional peloton is now simplifying its approach. Dr Hulse, I suspect, is a man who likes the new simplicity and clarity: 'There has been an increasing realisation that training had become gratuitously granular and detailed – the new paradigm is low/medium/high, of which "medium" is the most poorly defined.'

This new approach is echoed by elite coach Garth Fox, who also supports a more reductive approach to training zones: 'There are only three training zones that are physiologically valid. Low intensity (< 80 per cent of maximum heart rate [HR]), medium intensity (80–87 per cent of maximum HR), and hard (>87 per cent of maximum HR). These are anchored by blood lactate and respiratory changes that occur when we take an athlete from rest to maximal effort.'

Dr Hulse and coach Fox may arm-wrestle over the exact metrics, but the ethos is entirely congruent. I'll argue later that three levels are probably still one too many for most of us, by a factor of about one. When it comes to training levels and what fuels them, all roads necessarily lead eventually to a compound called adenosine triphosphate (ATP), the common denominator raw material that powers all of our muscular contractions and neural impulses. We do store a limited amount of ATP in our muscles, but the majority has to be synthesised in our mitochondria.

Low intensity training used to be referred to for decades as 'aerobic', but is now known as 'oxidative phosphorylation', which is much snappier. Garth puts a value on these training efforts as anything up to < 80% of our maximum heart rate. So, from the percentages above, a maximum HR of 162bpm would correspond to us being oxidative up to a heart rate of 162 × 80% = 130bpm. Oxidative not only relates to heart rate but also directly to what energy source we're relying upon to fuel our efforts – a combination of glucose and fatty acids, which is made into ATP in the mitochondria using oxygen. Provided we've consumed enough fatty acids and glucose (and we normally have), and we keep our exertion below 130bpm, we'll have an almost limitless precious ATP via the oxygen-fuelled bonfire in our mitochondria. Long, steady-state rides are mostly conducted in an oxidative or aerobic state. Working in an oxidative state is hugely efficient because it's so sustainable in the long term. Moreover it's no surprise that we feel comfortable in this state because of our evolved history of persistence hunting, where we may have had to walk or jog for hours or days to secure our prey. As a rule of thumb, if you are riding at 80 per cent of your maximum heart rate, you will be able to hold a conversation with someone else in the bunch.

Moving up a notch to medium training intensity, and still assuming our maximum heart rate of 162bpm, we're now working in a range of 130bpm to around 140bpm (possibly a little more). Casual conversation may just have become a little more challenging. Running on our 'medium' setting, we're now synthesising our vital ATP using a fast-acting process called glycolysis, which involves processing glycogen or glucose to provide quick energy. But once we blend from mainly oxidative into a glycolysis state we lose the ability to convert our more ubiquitous fatty acid stores in favour of the more relatively scarce glucose. The process of glycolysis doesn't happen in the mitochondria but within the cytosol, or intracellular fluid. This level of activity used to be referred to as 'anaerobic lactic' because it functions without oxygen and will produce increasing amounts of a substance called lactate as a by-product. Your body will, for a while at least, be able to keep you in equilibrium by processing lactate as you continue to work at an incrementally higher level. Inevitably there will come a time, if you keep increasing your work rate, where your body starts to lose the battle, and more lactate is being produced than you can re-metabolise. At this point, conversation generally becomes much more monosyllabic, and if you keep going you may start to feel an ache or tightness in your muscles. The term 'lactate threshold' is the last point of equilibrium, where your body is just managing to process as much lactate as it's producing.

Top of the tree is Dr Dave and Garth's hard (or high intensity) training level – which takes us from 87 per cent of our maximum HR all the way to our theoretical maximum of 162bpm. Previously known as 'anaerobic alactic' or 'without lactic', it's now referred to as utilising a 'phosphagen pathway'. This facilitates the rapid deployment of ATP and creatine for maximum power production over a very limited time. It is the quickest possible deployment of intense muscular contractions but can be sustained only while reserves of creatine phosphate exist within the muscle fibres themselves. This may be only tens of seconds. Road racers ply their trade via their ability to deploy and rebuild their stocks of creatine phosphate and skeletal muscle ATP. This is the rocket fuel that will launch you across a 30-second gap to the breakaway, or win you the race with a well-timed, all-out sprint coming out of the last corner – I get excited just thinking about it! Good road racers, and especially criterium riders, are masters of keeping an internal audit of their creatine phosphate and ATP stocks via the sensations in their legs and in their lungs. It's as addictive as any chemical ever invented by any pharmacist. It's a feeling that you never forget – that split-second perfect explosion, without pain or necessarily a sensation of being particularly more out of breath, since it operates without oxygen or lactate. Until you come crashing back to reality when the afterburners flame out.

The reason that Dr Hulse's and coach Fox's three training levels are a good starting point is because they perfectly overlay with what we objectively know about humans and their physiological (respiratory/ blood) changes as we increase their exercise workloads. The only speculative part is how it applies to an individual – hence Dr Hulse's caveat around the medium intensity training level in particular. Since the medium level of activity is the 'most poorly defined', it becomes clear that this is the level I'm proposing should be dropped – it's too nebulous from one rider to the next, since one person's glycolysis is another person's oxidative phosphorylation, so to speak. It's also quite ill-defined as to how long an individual can ride in a purely glycolysis state – five minutes, half an hour, two hours?

Professional cyclists generally know as much about their bodies and blood values as NASA astronauts, so it's easier for them to be accurate about how they structure their training. For the rest of us, there are a few more markers that we can look at to see if we want to add them to our toolbox.

The first one was the 'gold standard test' from 20 years ago, and this was the one we all talked about, although we never really understood what it was – we just knew it could predict how far you could go in our beloved sport. Above 75 and you could be an elite, 60–67 was a good amateur, 50–60 and you were an also-ran – yes, the dreaded test was the VO_2 Max. This was a lab ramp test of how much volume (V) of oxygen (O_2) your body could use as a proportion of your body weight in kilograms in one minute. It was an awful test because you had to go from tickover to redline in ramped increments, while wearing a Hannibal Lecter mask, generally with people watching, your cycling credentials and future landscape dangling by a fine thread, all administered by a badly dressed man with a clipboard. The day we did our VO_2 Max test, our teammate, Warrick Spence, scored 82. The sports scientist doing the testing was so excited he could barely be bothered to test Jules and myself. He had found his rough diamond shining in a pile of gravel. Jules and I predictably scored poorly – I was 54, I think, and Jules a little bit better. But we were donkeys fortunate to be sharing a stable with a pure thoroughbred. We were both also around 40 years old when we were tested (Warrick was in his 20s), working long hours starting Cyclefit and not training and racing as much as we used to. VO_2 doesn't care – the also-ran prognosis was clear. Cycling folklore has it that the enigmatic Sean Kelly had a similar experience when he rode for the Dutch PDM team in the late 1980s. This was a time when sports science was moving in to cycling and had started VO_2 testing of entire teams (for what end, I suspect nobody knew). The tale, maybe apocryphal, is that Kelly delivered a very poor VO_2 result and walked away from the test rig, not at all perturbed, when he was challenged by the team doctors and sports scientists as to how he produced spectacular race results with such a poor score. His reply: 'Your machine doesn't measure suffering, does it?'

God, how I hope that story is true! It's why I started cycling and why bike racing has transfixed me for decades, both as a spectator and racer.

Was Kelly's mumbled question rhetorical, or was he challenging the scientists' emerging worldview of subjugating sport to a calculation?

I can't really recommend a VO_2 Max test to anyone reading this book because I don't know what you'll do with the result, or how it will help you enjoy your riding more. It didn't help us when we were racing, and it wouldn't help us now. What we can say, with every confidence, is that if you're currently cycling regularly, then your current VO_2 Max is probably around 70 per cent higher than your age-matched sedentary contemporaries. VO_2 Max was the bragging rights metric of 20–30 years ago, and most of us had no idea what to usefully do with the number, other than compare it to Greg LeMond's 92.5.

Onto the 21st-century bragging metric, and one we've all probably heard of – functional threshold power (FTP), which we touched on in chapter 3. In its simplest terms, FTP is the highest average power you can sustain for one hour. More recently, FTP has also come to include a 20-minute figure, because an hour at sustainable maximum was difficult for many people. It's called 'functional' because it's meant to have a real-world application.

Before power meters were invented we used to routinely complete FTP tests, except we called them time trials – most typically 16 or 40km. Coincidentally, a '10' would take about 20 minutes and a '25' about an hour. We were doing FTPs every week before we even knew they existed. As an aside, as we got fitter and stronger progressing through the season, our average speed for a 25 would get closer to our average speed for a 10. FTP is thought to be reasonably well correlated to lactate threshold.

Incidentally FTP was devised by Dr Andrew Coggan – a very clever and innovative American physiologist (and renowned time triallist). I wonder if there was any cognitive bias at play here? FTP has become the new benchmark for all structured training. Every two-wheeled athlete and all of their coaches will have one eye on it. But is it always appropriate? It's certainly more applicable to the real world than an entirely abstract VO_2

number – what were we supposed to do with 54 mL/kg/min, except perhaps retire depressed? It doesn't help me train or tell me what I'm capable of or how to improve. It's just a badge to wear and a flag to hoist unless you know how to professionally decode it. At least FTP theoretically shows us how far and fast we can ride for 20 minutes (or one hour) should we want to. As a sustainable power metric run in controlled conditions it's also reasonably easy to repeat, and therefore monitor fitness improvement or decline. But does it have any intrinsic value in and of itself?

It has intrinsic value only if your cycling goal is to ride as fast as you can for 20 minutes or an hour and then collapse in a sweaty heap. Remember, we're highly adaptive organisms and will become incrementally better at whatever training stress or stimulus we subject our bodies to. Strangely enough, FTP doesn't have much application for the kind of racing that I used to do – shortish road races and fast criteriums. In fact, as regards the latter, Dr Stephens points out: 'You ride a criterium and your watts are either at 70 or 700, hardly ever at your FTP.' This isn't to say that having a high FTP isn't an indication of general aerobic fitness, but it won't help you win a criterium, where a 30-second squirt of power is the holy grail. Look at Mark Cavendish – I'm pretty sure he was only ever fleetingly interested in his FTP because it wasn't the metric he needed to measure to prepare for sprints. Equally, if you want to take part in the Trans-Continental Race or Paris–Brest–Paris, you would be ill-advised to ride anywhere near your FTP because these efforts would be fuelled by the ephemeral process of glycosis – your fuel of choice should be glucose and fatty acids metabolised in the mitochondria in an aerobic environment. Dr Baker adds: 'FTP doesn't represent anything, it's a contentious subject, it's something that's routinely used to set training levels but it's not a measure of anything physiological.'

The timescales set do seem incredibly arbitrary – why is it 20 minutes or an hour and not an hour and 11 minutes? But of course FTP does have validity if you're an athlete training for the midlife hour record or a midlife time triallist whose aspiration is to break 40km in an hour.

At that point it is right that this metric, which we now call FTP, has specific application, regardless of what aspect of physiology it is measuring or approximating.

There are several other potential problems with using FTP as your training lodestar, quite apart from its arbitrariness. The biggest is that FTP isn't a ratchet and there will be a moment, regardless of what you do, when it will plateau or even start declining. Will you be quite so interested in tracking your static or diminishing FTP as you are your steady improvement? If you really are dispassionately interested in data, then your answer must be yes.

Quite possibly the lowest-tech training device ever devised is the rate of perceived exertion (RPE). It's cheaper than either a heart rate monitor or a power meter because it's entirely free. We all use RPE when we train, but recently technology has tended to shuffle our valuable introspection to the bottom of the deck. RPE was introduced by a Swedish psychologist, Dr Gunnar Borg, in the 1950s and is sometimes referred to as the Borg Scale. The scale runs from 6 to 20, with clearly delineated waypoints: 6 means no apparent exertion at all, such as reading a book or lying down, whereas 20 means maximal exertion. Borg started his scale at 6 rather than 1 because he wanted to make it approximately applicable to heart rate, by multiplying the numbers on the scale by 10. No exertion at all would be $6 \times 10 = 60$bpm, and at the other end of the scale, maximal exertion would be $20 \times 10 = 200$bpm. Although this sounds a little on the high side for most us midlifers, I do know of at least one 55-year-old hummingbird out there. So this is the Borg Scale:

- 6 – No exertion at all
- 7 – Extremely light
- 8
- 9 – Very light
- 10

- 11 – Light
- 12
- 13 – Somewhat hard
- 14
- 15 – Hard
- 16
- 17 – Very hard
- 18
- 19 – Extremely hard
- 20 – Maximal exertion

Paralysis by analysis

'Paralysed' is Dr Baker's phrase, not mine, but perfectly encapsulates the risk of data overload that comes with taking everything too seriously and allowing the analysis and sports science to overtake the sport. I have friends, who if their power meter fails, would rather not ride at all – for · them, the ride didn't exist if it wasn't recorded. We all need to find the right recipe of technology and training structure that suits our aspirations and personalities. At one end of the spectrum you have my chaotic seat-of-pants, ride-how-you-feel vibe, and revel in the consequences (I'm almost certainly looking at the past with sepia-tinted binoculars and I probably had way more bad racing days than good). And at the other end of the spectrum, an adherence to a micro-planned, metric-driven, yellow-brick road to incremental improvement and full personal potential achievement.

I think that you should take a structured, data-driven, technological approach to your riding if you like facts and figures and find them fascinating and intrinsically fun, regardless of whether they are personally moving in a positive direction or not. Also take the data-driven route if your performance has plateaued or deteriorated and you're interested to know why. Dr Baker relates the experience of a client who had miscalculated their FTP by a whopping 20 per cent, resulting in them inadvertently constantly training too close to their threshold and becoming a somewhat poor and very fatigued 'endurance athlete' (endurance was their stated goal) – 'essentially they were 40 watts over in every training session'. By doing some diligent diagnostic work and resetting their levels, Dr Baker was able to dial back their efforts to a place that would help them improve their long-term aerobic base, without embedding fatigue. You could potentially make all those moves yourself without a coach, power meter or heart rate monitor. But sometimes it helps when you're in a hole if someone else tells you to stop digging, and at the same time provides the evidentiary data behind their apparent wisdom. Lastly, use data if you're riding at that level where tiny improvements make all the difference. You don't have to be professional, of course, but you are riding to a quantifiable goal where tiny, perceptible improvements could be the difference between gold and silver. Dr Stephens says: 'There's quite a lot about training that's just doing what you feel. And maybe the last five per cent is to do with very structured training and peaking and tapering and that kind of stuff.'

Do what you feel

Interestingly, even in elite sports circles there's a move to make training more empathic and simpler – less prescriptive and more athlete-led. In the world of elite running some researcher-coaches have resorted to philosophers to guide them on the best approach to getting the best out of their athletes. Specifically, French philosopher Michel Foucault, whose work (and I summarise) centred around the concept that excessively rigid structures tend to make people unhelpfully passive, feeling like they lack control and self-expression. Clearly not helpful in the multi-dimensional chess game of road racing, where dynamic decision-making and athletic performance are crucial (although Team Sky had their spirit-flattening moments). The Foucauldian model, in contrast, is to encourage the athlete to take more control and ownership of how they feel and how their training should be conducted in any one session. The coach may just ask the athlete to train how they feel on any given day rather than prescribe (see how we use medical words) a set-piece agenda of intervals. Apparently the athletes being coached under the Foucault 'do what you feel' philosophy often perform at a higher level of intensity and effort than if they are being micro-directed. I was a Foucauldian before my time.

I was somewhat bought down to earth by one of my oldest and closest friends, Dr Peter Atterton, Professor of Philosophy at SDSU in San Diego, published Foucault scholar (and road cyclist): 'I don't really think it has much to do with Foucault. Seems like one of those attempts to introduce an exotic species that isn't native to the place where it is introduced but instead has been deliberately transported to the new location by human activity. It usually ends badly.'

Peter may not like the contrived overlay of Foucault onto the athletics track or elite sports science, but the idea that individual athletes could take more responsibility for their own development, based on how they feel, is surely compelling. And this approach resonates with Cyclefit's own approach to working with professional cyclists as individuals (as opposed to part of a team – when we were working within the team structure, it was logistically necessary to give out slots for road and TT fits for each rider through the week. And then by definition there had to be a prescribed fitting methodology and procedure, so we didn't overrun). Now we're not contracted to a single team, instead we work with individuals from many teams, who consult with us from time to time about any issues or questions they may have that relate to their cycling biomechanics. It's a far superior dynamic – they are rightly in control of the session and will elicit the information and opinion that they need to improve their comfort, efficiency and function. The Foucauldian approach to bike fitting. Sorry, Peter.

But I don't know what I feel

Taking control, or doing what you feel, does not necessarily mean flying solo or 'barefoot' cycling. Just as our clients don't have to know everything about cycling biomechanics – although it certainly helps if they gain some knowledge – you're not expected to know everything about training and the physiological systems you're accessing to gain fitness. But it certainly does help for us to understand our own bodies, have the intuition to set realistic goals and then act rationally to achieve them. Dr Baker has 10 million kilometres of accumulated training data from a mixture of professional and amateur clients, from over the years. One of the fascinating trends is that 'World Tour guys ride over a whole season at around 62–65 per cent of their maximum. In contrast, if you look at the slowest guys, they are at 80 per cent of their maximum over their whole season – which is counterintuitive.'

Us older and less fit midlife cyclists are, as a group, riding harder and faster, relative to our maximum, than the top-ranked professionals in the world. And we're holding down jobs, and trying to be great parents and partners. Dr Baker's data can't lie, it's just data. His amateur clients (that's you and me) are closer to fatigue and nearer to being overtrained than the professionals who ride for a living and race nine months of the year all around the world! That statement was genuinely worthy of an exclamation mark. And underpinning this startling mismatch is a fundamental misunderstanding about how the human body works, and therefore improves.

Many amateurs perpetually train and ride in what Dr Baker calls a 'whirlwind of doom' where an overestimation and obsession with an FTP (an abstract number in itself) means that we tend to set our training levels too high and, as a consequence, are training the wrong systems and incrementally embedding fatigue that we then struggle to shake off if we're older, because our hormonal responses are less responsive and dynamic – is this ringing any bells?

Going long!

Drs Hulse and Baker, and coach Fox, all go out of their way to remind us that cycling (other than sprinting on a track) is fundamentally an endurance sport – and endurance is what we're best at compared to other animals. Recent studes have even suggested that the drive to efficiency and therefore endurance is what selectively drove us towards bipedalism. We may not be super-sprinters compared to other big mammals (I can't think of a single one we can beat in a short burst), but we can go seriously long, which meant that we could subsistence hunt much larger prey than ourselves over multiple days.

But what constitutes endurance? Dr Baker says: 'Endurance has to mean aerobic – which is determined by the strength and ability of the heart, and then the ability of the blood, to transport fuel to the muscles, and the muscles to then use that fuel.'

Aerobic, as we know, is a cipher for functioning within an oxidative state – using fatty acids and glucose as fuel with oxygen, which is metabolised in our muscle's mitochondria to produce energy. It's our long-burn, sustainable state. Our most important goal as endurance athletes surely has to be to increase our oxidative or aerobic performance window, to become better at producing more power but at the same time staying oxidative/aerobic. We need to become lean, long-burn machines and the only way to achieve this is to ride at this specific level – remember that we're highly adaptable creatures and our bodies will change and improve based on specific repeated stresses.

And this is where power meters and heart rate monitors can help – if we make them truly our servants and not our masters. They can help us become more honest with ourselves about our own performance and how we feel. The best way to use a heart rate monitor or a power meter is as a bandwidth limiter. If you're oxidative all the way up to 135bpm or 160 watts, then that's where the majority of your riding should be in order to improve as an endurance athlete. If you're working at this level, then you're the recipient of a cascade of positive physiological responses, including increasing the mitochondria in your muscles. Every time you go above this level, you're having to use enzymes to break down the excess lactate. Dr Baker's coach's eye view: 'If you feel good on an endurance ride, go longer, not harder. Going harder is risky. Going longer is safe. It's the same with intervals – if you feel good, do an extra rep or two, but don't increase the power.'

If you don't have a power meter or a heart rate monitor, you can use the RPE, or Borg Scale. If you want to be a great endurance athlete, most of your training should be at a level where you can have a fairly normal conversation with the person next to you, or sing a whole verse of a song without stopping and gasping for breath. On a Borg Scale this would still be quite low – maybe 12 or 13, where 6 is lying on a bed reading a book and 20 is full effort. You'll know if you're ceasing to work aerobically (or, in an oxidative state) because you'll start panting or gasping if you try to sing out loud or tell anything more than a quick one-line joke. This is because when enough lactate has accumulated in your system, your brain will automatically preference breathing over talking, in an attempt to clear CO_2 out of your system and bring you back into aerobic equilibrium. It's worth pointing out that recovery from endurance rides is also easier than recovery from intense interval sessions, where the fatigue tends to be embedded deeper into our physiological and muscular skeletal systems. As Dr Baker puts it: 'The "hours of power" approach tends to make you more tired as the quality of your sessions declines. Ergo, if you're less tired you tend to miss less training days, which has to be good because fundamentally endurance equals volume.'

Is this where the old school, my chaotic school and the new-data school intersect? We all seem to be saying the same thing. That to build yourself into a persistence (or endurance) hunter you need to train yourself to be a hyper-efficient aerobic machine, ruthless at scavenging sustainable fuel stores at as high-power outputs as possible. It isn't a high FTP that will get you round a big day in the mountains, it's a high-functioning aerobic system. If you've inadvertently trained the wrong system by going too deep and too hard, you'll be producing excess lactate and utilising precious glycogen stores too quickly, which in turn will make a fit-for-purpose refuelling strategy very difficult. Dr Baker thinks that most amateur riders function at only 60 per cent of their theoretical aerobic (oxidative) capacity due to training incorrectly – mostly from riding too much at too high a level. You need to be a fast tortoise before you can become even a slow hare.

Both coach Fox and Dr Baker agree that the majority of riding should be steady-state to increase our oxidative capacity – as much as 80–90 per cent of our training load. We have to learn to be efficient before we can learn to be fast. But even as midlife cyclists we can gain a huge amount of benefit from the correct dose of intense interval training.

Controversially, I'm going to suggest a few midlife amendments to current training orthodoxy. The first is that we drop all the other stratas of training, other than low intensity (LIT) and high intensity (HIT) training. We'll define LIT as anything below aerobic threshold, which coach Fox recommends could be as high as 70–80 per cent of maximum heart rate, but thinks is actually better executed at around 60–70 per cent of maximum. Dr Baker agrees with this and adds the context that 'it's almost impossible to go too low' for LIT or oxidative training, meaning that the most important principle to observe is that you must actually be oxidative, which you won't be if you go too high.

You could use a heart rate monitor and use a percentage of your highest recent recorded heart rate or you could use the RPE/Borg Scale and the 'sing-a-verse' methodology (which I prefer, incidentally). It's important to note that riding in an oxidative state involves metabolising fatty acids as a fuel source, which could be important if you're also trying to manage weight as well as gain fitness.

Anything above LIT, is by definition in our binary training model, HIT. If you're using the RPE/Borg Scale, LIT is anything below 14, HIT is 15–20. Both Dr Baker and coach Fox suggest no more than one or two sessions a week, and how you configure them can be the result of your own imagination. It could be hill repeats (not imaginative but can be effective) or Dr Baker's suggestion: 'There's gold in 8–10-minute efforts in the 105–110 per cent of FTP range. The goal is to do *lots* of reps, say 4–6. If you hold power steady, then your heart rate won't quite hit your maximum. So you can rest up a bit, and repeat again.'

Remember, Dr Baker is going out of his way to point out that if you feel good, you should *not* increase the intensity, meaning no more watts or a higher heart rate, but instead add in a rep or two. Going too deep or too hard will increase the required recovery time and may lead to fatigue. If you assume your real (not inflated FTP) is 250, then your hard sessions using the Dr Baker algorithm will be 250 × 105–110% × 4–6 (8–10 minute) reps. This means that you'll be working at between 262 and 275 watts during those 8–10 minute reps. This isn't going bonkers and sending your systems haywire – it's a controlled elevation of training stimulus. Coach Fox's thoughts on the subject of sensible restraint are these: 'The important aspect (and the part that amateur athletes have enormous difficulty in executing well) is that only about 10–20 per cent maximum of training time needs to be here. This can be done as one or two harder interval sessions per week, but not more as that just leads to plateauing sooner [rather] than later. It really should be no more complicated than that. In fact, I would hypothesise the opposite.'

Dr Baker and coach Fox are united in the opinion that us amateurs – especially more time-constrained masters athletes, because we want to optimise our limited time – mostly train too hard, when we should be working in an oxidative state and not incorporating too many intense interval sessions. Essentially, we're over-revving ourselves into aerobic inefficiency or, even worse, embedding fatigue in our bodies by riding too often, too close to threshold, and not leaving sufficient recovery time between training sessions. We're not only burning the candle at both ends, we're then taking a blow torch to it to make sure it's dead.

Recovery 101

Apparently many of us veteran athletes have either forgotten the main principles of training and recovery (or maybe we didn't absorb them properly in the first place).

For the purpose of recap, we build additional fitness when we're resting, not when we're training. This is called 'supercompensation'. This is a response to a training stimulus that's greater than your body is generally used to. You'll then recover from that stimulus or training dose, and because we're adaptive, or plastic, creatures, your body will modify the necessary structures (muscles, cardiovascular system, etc) so it can cope with the anticipated extra physical load next time. This is broken into four stages – we start with our initial fitness, then move to the training stimulus or event. After the event we're tired and depleted and need to recover. Only after recovery is complete do we move into the vital adaptive supercompensation stage. Imagine you have a big event like L'Étape or La Marmotte. You start the morning with a certain fitness level, then subject all your body's systems to a massive and probably unprecedented training dose. Immediately after the event your body will want to recover and heal – your strength and performance reserves, at this point, will be way below the level that you started with directly prior to the event. Even if a mysterious and, it has to be said, slightly sadistic benefactor, offered you £5,000 to get straight back on your bike and ride the course in reverse, you would (and should) refuse. Your body is at its weakest and least capable at this point – if you decided to try getting back on your bike, it would almost certainly end in painful failure and possibly longer-lasting problems. Once your body has recovered, however, fuelled by good food, extra hydration, essential electrolytes and minerals, and most importantly rest and sleep, it enters the supercompensation phase where the strengthening process takes place. How long that whole process lasts is hard to predict, because it will depend on so many variables, such as level of prior fitness, training dose, age, nutrition, hydration and any underlying physical issues. But the principle is clear – training introduces a stimulus that significantly weakens us in the short term. But the training dose triggers adaptations in the body that will make us incrementally stronger if – and only if – we allow the body to recover and rest properly. On a physiological level, the actual building process of fitness and strength improvement occurs when we are resting and not when we are training.

For some people it would mean that, should you ride the same event a week later, you would be substantially faster and more composed. For others, a week wouldn't be nearly long enough, while a lucky handful would be flying by Tuesday. The best people at predicting these training/peaking outcomes are people like Dr Baker and coach Fox, who have files full of data on clients they have guided through big events.

Even though my own training was chaotic, I had an innate understanding of this process. I knew very well the specific racing doses that my body needed to improve coming into the season. Even though the efforts in the early races were harder than I was acclimatised to and therefore quite unpleasant in the moment, I made sure that I was fuelled, rested and ready for the process. The kind of efforts that worked well for me were short, explosive criteriums where you're going from tickover to redline and back to tickover, what felt like hundreds of times for over an hour. A handful of these kinds of events after a long winter just riding quietly doing easy miles with friends was enough. My body recovered and supercompensated to tolerate a new and elevated level of function. The next level was peaking, which I was never very good at. I could have set my watch by the decline. By the end of June I would hit a week or two of rare form – those lovely moments, we all have them, when it's literally impossible to hurt yourself, because your body has become so free-revving and responsive. It was like finding a secret entrance to a gold mine – deep seams of enriched vitality and energy that appear to spool out endlessly into the future. Except they don't, and in my experience, what I thought of as new equilibrium was in fact a precarious knife-edge that I could balance on for only a fleeting instant. Sports science has come a long way, but as far as I know, has found no method of turning the peak into a new plateau.

Overtraining syndrome (OTS)

A word on overtraining syndrome. This sounds like a harmless sounding phrase that almost connotes a commendable work ethic, but in my experience 'overtraining' is little more than a euphemism for something highly unpleasant and disruptive. I have had a few clients over the last couple of decades who have made themselves severely ill with overtraining, and at least one of them now has permanent physical damage. At its most serious, overtraining is a recognised medical condition and is treated as such by a physician.

Drs Kreher and Schwartz define it in their 2012 paper as 'a maladapted response to excessive exercise without adequate rest, resulting in perturbations of multiple body systems (neurologic, endocrinologic, immunologic) coupled with mood changes.'

Overtraining switches from being an abstract concept to an actual syndrome when central fatigue and overreach get so embedded that your body stops reacting positively to training stimulus and now starts to react negatively. You could have negative symptoms such as low mood, insomnia, weight loss, sore muscles and loss of interest in training, as well as other issues like poor sleep, irritability, restlessness and slow heart rate (bradycardia).

There's ongoing research into why you may be able to tolerate a high training load for a while but then succumb to a negative cascade. It could be that there's a sudden additional and unacknowledged stress on the system which tips you over the edge, such as an emotional problem, a virus or an allergy. Or it could be a cumulative problem because your training or nutrition strategy were flawed and your body can no longer tolerate being in deficit.

One of the theories is that OTS is triggered by excess inflammation or 'cytokine hypothesis'. Cytokines are tiny proteins important in cell signalling, which help regulate our immune response and inflammation. Cytokines are helpful when they are marshalling cells towards an injury or infection. But it is thought cytokines can be harmful when there is an over-reaction and the cytokine activity is inappropriately high, and causes excess inflammation. The worst effects of Covid-19 are thought to be caused by a cytokine storm. OTS and the long-term illness that often follows is thought to be linked to an over-reaction of our immune system, leading to an excess of inflammation.

Normal muscular activity associated with hard training and tissue renewal causes local inflammation, but in OTS this somehow tips over into a more serious inflammatory response that affects the whole body, possibly due to insufficient recovery or another contributory factor. Left unchecked, this can become a more systemic and chronic inflammation.

Every sports physician and physiologist we've ever consulted went out of their way to highlight that veteran athletes need longer to recover between sessions to improve. Without adequate recovery the possibility of OTS is very real, so we must be careful. I have seen it in the most driven and determined clients. On at least one occasion it was due to overexertion in a particular event, associated with excess heat and a poorly executed hydration strategy. It wasn't their fault that the event ran out of water and electrolytes, but it was their fault (though understandable) that they pressed on in 38-degree heat until they collapsed. At that point they could no longer absorb water orally and needed medical treatment. The universal physiological strain this puts on any athlete, but especially a midlife athlete, is far from trivial. This particular individual took many months to recover to a full training programme and I suspect their performance was permanently compromised. Exercise is meant to be healthy and help us to live better lives with higher physical and cognitive function. OTS is a serious illness with occasional far-reaching consequences. We generally get to know our clients over a number of years and it's always a particular concern when they have the same cough for a few weeks or months yet still push through a big training block. We gently try referring them to their GP or someone like Dr Hulse for some more structured and informed advice. They generally lose weight, look gaunt, and exude low mood and fatigue. Often, they are distracted and lack focus. The knee, back or foot issue they want us to deal with is just a distraction or, at least, of secondary importance. Every mile they now ride is embedding further local and systemic damage. When we voice our concerns, we commonly get the same response – a cough, an 'ahem', and a vaguely embarrassed 'Yeah, I know, I just need to get through this block.'

This is the point when the client needs someone else – a coach or a physician – to protect them from themselves. If they were referred to any consultant the first prescription would be rest and recovery, followed by a stripping out of all hard efforts and high intensity. They have ignored every signpost and are on their way to potentially serious problems. Athletes, and especially cyclists, are mostly a self-selecting group – we're drawn to the sport because of the work ethic, incremental improvement and love of the hard miles. And more equals better, right? Except it doesn't when you're entrenching fatigue and possible illness.

Midlife performance – our top tips

We're not usually fans of these kinds of lists, but on this topic some quick tips are a good idea:

1. Keep it simple. Don't overcomplicate your training or get 'paralysis by analysis'. Our binary model of LIT and HIT is all most of us need. Stick to the rules – 80–90 per cent of your sessions should be training your oxidative systems to be more efficient.

2. Don't get obsessed with wearing FTP as a badge. Use your real FTP number to set realistic training stratas. Set these too high, and you just make your body very good at producing lactate – not helpful for an endurance athlete.

3. Use the heart rate monitor and/or power meter as limiters to make sure you don't overshoot training zones.

4   Remember heart monitors are notorious for having a lag – don't rely on them for accuracy during intense intervals, as you may over-rev.

5   Have only one or two HIT sessions per week. Go long rather than deep. These sessions should comprise only around 10 per cent of your training load.

6   And on the 'go long' subject, if you're feeling great, remember Dr Baker's advice and avoid going deep. Never go to 20 on the Borg Scale or keep bouncing off your heart rate maximum – it will only make recovery harder and longer. How about setting a rule that you always stay three per cent lower than your maximum heart rate – that's what we do at Cyclefit.

7   Ward off sarcopenia. You lose muscle faster than you lose aerobic condition – look at Dr Stephens, still matching the times he set as a 48-year-old a decade on. Drop a bike session for resistance training – this will also help with bone density and weight loss (muscle requires more energy than fat).

8   Are you the kind of person who gets obsessed and fixated? Get a coach to channel your work ethic in a constructive way and be that voice of reason on your shoulder.

9   If you're a Captain Chaos (my hand is up), maybe get a coach to add some structure to your training diet so you can see what you're really capable of.

10   Don't ignore injury symptoms. Your bike fit will probably change a little every year and niggles will become chronic injuries if you don't catch them rapidly.

11   Avoid OTS. At best this is disruptive – costing you months or even years of riding time. At worst, it has lifelong consequences. Sometimes the smartest thing you can do is go home. You're halfway up Mont Ventoux, it's 40 degrees, you've no water and you don't feel well? Take a step back – you have a full life and responsibilities off your bike.

12 Build up slowly. Dr Stephens made a point of saying that this is what has changed in his training approach as he has got older: 'I ride nearly every day of the week, but what I'm careful about is not to rapidly ramp it up.'

13 Remember that amateur veteran athletes tend to work at a proportionally higher rate than professional cyclists. Go slow to speed up. Avoid embedding structural fatigue.

14 Do something else! As you get older you should probably bring in something else. If you don't like yoga or pilates, think about a complimentary sport, such as paddleboarding, swimming, running – all three require spinal extension rather than the flexed position we tend to adopt on the bike. My personal favourite for cyclists is paddleboarding because it works on everything we're notoriously bad at – core strength, balance, upper body strength, good posture, and so on. Plus, it's fun and aerobic or anerobic – sorry, 'oxidative' or 'phosphagen pathway'. There's one school of thought that 'training boredom' is a component of overtraining syndrome. Variety will keep you physically and mentally nimble and rejuvenated.

15 Get proper rest and recovery – you'll need more of both as you get older. You'll not be the exception, so accept it as a part of getting older – you cannot fight your hormones. You should review your training mix regularly to ensure that you're building in quality rest and recovery. Every single one of the medical professionals that we spoke to went out of their way to reinforce this.

16 Keep your indoor cycling sessions to a minimum. Although this sounds controversial, there are good reasons:

• Posture/technique. We tend to ride in poorer body positions on static trainers – we stand less, use gears that are too high, have poorer saddle stability and contact, and load up the arms, neck and shoulders.

- Environmental. Indoor cycling is often associated with hot, sweaty rooms, where it's easy to overheat and get dehydrated.
- Technique. Training outside is palpably better for your balance, riding skills and cognition. It's also better for your general mood and mental health. There's no point training indoors all winter and then descending the mountains in the summer, at a slower pace than you climb because of a lack of confidence and skills.
- Training integrity. Riding inside on static trainers often encourages us to ride above our sensible and recommended zones. This lessens the training effect and negatively affects recovery, especially if you're virtually competing with other people – you're effectively subsuming your own training session into theirs. However, you could make a static bike session one of your HITs during the week.
- Abstraction. Just as running machines aren't the best training for running, so static trainers aren't the best way to build a cyclist. Let the randomness and chaos of the road or trail build a deeper resilience and flexibility of fitness.
- Barefoot cycling. Once a month go barefoot – no computer, no heart rate monitor. Ride entirely on a Foucaldian 'how you feel' basis, and use the RPE/Borg Scale to measure effort levels. The session will be mentally liberating and refreshing, and also maintain your vital introspection RPE skills. Afterwards, you could use Strava to retrospectively interpret the ride data.
- Make sure you read chapters 7 and 8, where we have a few things to say about alcohol and sleep, among other things.

There are a thousand books out there that can instruct you, with copious graphs, how to slice, ever more thinly, the training sausage. But it can be beautifully simple. Train very easy when your body is in recovery, or tired, or when you just feel like it. Train hard when your body is supercharged with rest and good nutrition, to the point where you're almost literally fizzing with middle-aged vitality and enthusiasm. And don't confuse the two by going 'quite hard' most of the time, which is the big bear trap for amateurs. The data clearly shows that amateur cyclists spend more time closer to their theoretical red line than the professionals. This tends to make us fantastic lactate production factories but singularly not great endurance athletes. The negative spiral of fatigue, irritability and poor performance awaits all of us if we misplace a great work ethic over wisdom and common sense. And this syndrome progressively gets more acute as we get older and it takes us longer to recover from harder efforts. In the old world, we would put in that extra hill repeat, because if you didn't, the competition damn well would. In the new world, maybe you keep that last rep in your back pocket as you take the long, slow, meandering route home listening to the bird song and depowering your sympathetic nervous system back to its standby mode? Maybe you arrive home relaxed in a parasympathetic state, your body already preparing to refuel and recover. Go long.

5

BIKES, BIKE FIT AND BIOMECHANICS

Nobody hates the 'J' word more than I, where 'J' stands for 'journey' and is normally preceded by the word 'personal' and includes details of a yoga retreat or week-long silence in a monastic cell. But it's clear that as midlife cyclists, we have to acknowledge life's arc and the changes that are inevitably happening within our bodies and minds as we get older. And while it's true that exercise, and especially high-level exercise, does bring huge physiological and cognitive benefits and protection, it's also true that we can run the risk of having too much of a good thing, which can result in injury and illness. As we've learned from chapter 2, the bicycle inherently has so much to recommend it to midlife athletes in terms of joint protection and muscle trauma, compared to running, rugby and squash, etc. But the legacy of the fundamentals of cycling biomechanics which the Victorians kindly bequeathed us, and which was eternally and some (OK, I) would say unhelpfully preserved in aspic by the UCI, creates challenges that need to be continually considered if you want to stay healthy, fit and meet your goals as you age. In short, human beings didn't evolve to ride bikes, whatever the Victorian gentlemen inventors thought or intended at the time. In this chapter we explore the practical aspects of the relationship between the bike and the midlife body and how it can be preserved, or even improved, as we elegantly age.

In chapter 2 we interlocked Alex Fugallo's hypermobile–stiffness spectrum with Phil Burt's micro-adjuster–macro-absorber spectrum. And I invited you to think of where you sit on both. Are you a princess with her pea on the bike? Or can you ride anything, anywhere and never feel a moment of pain or discomfort? Do you struggle with flexibility? Or are you naturally abundant in your joint muscle ranges and always have been? You should have an idea where you sit on those two scales (no self-delusion, please – it won't help anyone). In this chapter, we'll look in more detail at the biomechanical interface between the human and the bicycle and how this relationship can change over time.

The perfect cycling body

Before we look at what can go wrong in the body-to-bike relationship department, it might be interesting to think about the perfect cycling physique. In our opinion anyway. Bear in mind that the bike is, by definition, at least to start with, entirely symmetrical – cycling therefore rewards symmetry, or at the very least one needs to know where someone exhibits asymmetry, to potentially intervene with a compensation. For example, we've worked with many athletes, including professional cyclists, who exhibit a spinal scoliosis – an S-shape in the spine, when viewed from the back. None of us are robots of course (one of our favourite aphorisms in the fit studio), so all of us have little kinks and irregularities in our morphology, but it's a question of extent. An extreme scoliosis can take the head, shoulders, hands, arms and even hips and legs out of alignment. An extreme bike position can exacerbate the asymmetry of a scoliosis over time, often resulting in pain and poor performance. Someone who exhibits a significant scoliosis will almost certainly be a micro-adjuster who finds it hard to produce high power outputs in an aggressive drop bar position. They'll feel like their body is fighting the position and/or that their head is shifted off to one side of the bike. They'll almost certainly feel much better when they are standing up out of the saddle when they are climbing or generating big torque loads through the pedals. When you're trapped by a machine that's micro-prescribing both contact-points and movement dynamics, a scoliosis is potentially more of a problem than when running, where the body is inherently freer to express itself. That's not to say that someone with a scoliosis shouldn't cycle, they should, but it's also true to say that as you ride harder and longer, it's likely that you'll be making good friends with your bike fitter and osteopath, to make sure that your bike set-up reflects your body as best as it can. We've worked with more than one professional cyclist who had a moderate or significant scoliosis, so it's perfectly possible to function at the very highest level with this kind of asymmetry. However, I personally think it's very difficult to maintain performance over time without a detailed physical therapy regime and constant position and equipment review. So, the first step to building the perfect cycling specimen is being symmetrical.

The second step is flexibility. You don't need to be a yoga teacher to be a great cyclist but you do need to be flexible enough (which begs an important question – are yoga teachers flexible because they're yoga teachers, or are they yoga teachers because they're flexible?). It's the same with great cyclists. We were attached to Trek Factory Racing (later Trek Segafredo) for four years and saw the changing of the guard from older, more established riders to newer and younger ones, with their refreshing thirst for self-knowledge and improvement. In the big training camps in December and January we would undertake a huge audit of the entire squad's physical conditioning and flexibility, called a 'functional movement screen' (FMS). It's a snapshot of one moment in time of your body's strengths, limitations and vulnerabilities.

We offer an FMS at Cyclefit, albeit on a more individualised basis. If you report pain in your hip, expect lots of range of motion tests in that area. If you present with an Achilles issue, you can expect a plethora of tests around the foot, calf and posterior chain, and so on. But with Trek Factory Racing the idea was to put the whole team through the same

FMS protocol to compare their flexibility, strength, symmetry, injury and pain presentation, at that moment in time. We would take this data collected during one week in early January and then use it as a valuable predictive tool for the coming season. For example, tightness in one hamstring in January could mean left-side lower-back pain in a Grand Tour. This meant that the team medics could build a programme of functional conditioning around a potential problem, to build in resilience for the rest of the season. The totality of our work with clients for two decades, combined with our controlled and data-driven audit approach with Trek, confirmed what we had long suspected – there's an almost binary relationship between flexibility and an athlete's ability to sustain aggressive riding positions. For example, Fabian Cancellara was always one of the most flexible riders in the squad, as well as being one of the most comprehensively conditioned in terms of his core and trunk strength. This gave him the ability to move from a standard road position to an aggressive aero position and yet still maintain within a couple of per cent of his sustainable road power. By contrast, other riders on the squad, who possibly struggled with flexibility (sometimes due to injury) could lose up to 23 per cent of their power moving between their road and aero positions. And bear in mind that 23 per cent for them is between 80 and 100 watts, far from trivial. We also see this binary relationship reflected in amateur cyclists and recreational cyclists and their ability to functionally achieve and hold aggressive positions on their bikes.

Flexibility is a slightly generic term – what do we mean by it, and what effect does it have on a cyclist's function?

Hip-in-flexion

Cycling is unique in the sense that we demand that the body functions with an acute femur-to-spine angle or hip-in-flexion, where the femur forms an acute angle with the spine at the top of the pedal-stroke. And the lower we maintain the torso, to lessen aerodynamic drag, the more acute this angle becomes. The only other sport I can think of that requires high torque with a closed hip is rowing – add this to the many reasons that rowers tend to move so seamlessly between the two sports. For professional cyclists, we look for around 130 degrees of hip-in-flexion for women, and at least 120 degrees for men. Hip-in-flexion means range of motion. It is the maximum spine to femur angle when the knee is pushed towards the chest (without boney or excessive soft-tissue impediment). The ability of the hip to function in flexion is essential because it ultimately dictates a person's sustainable torso/spine angle. If an athlete runs their bars very low (for example, 11cm of vertical drop from the saddle) but they have only 95 degrees of hip-in-flexion range (not uncommon), then the femur will hit a block at the top of the pedal stroke. This would probably result in the whole leg trying to deviate laterally (outwards) to avoid the restriction, or the body trying to bob and weave out of the way, or even compression into the delicate soft-tissue structures at the front of the hip (tendons, muscles). All of these adaptions are unhelpful, quite possibly under the conscious radar and almost certainly a longer-term route to under-performance or even injury.

The posterior chain

The posterior chain is the sum of the links that include calfs, hamstrings, glutes and muscles in your lower back – quadratus lumborum (QL). Tightness seems to be shared democratically around the posterior chain – so tight calf muscles are often a sign of tight hamstrings, and so on. This is important in cycling because tightness in the posterior chain exerts a negative control over your pelvis, meaning that it drags the pelvis back and down into a more passive and less dynamic posture. This in turn can lead to lower back pain over time as poor posture and poor core engagement becomes embedded. In short, as you try to rotate your pelvis forward to lower your torso and engage your glutes to produce more power, functional tightness in hamstrings and calves will be exerting forces in the opposite direction, which is wasteful and possibly painful.

Going back to Alex Fugallo's hypermobile–stiffness spectrum, it's our opinion that if you want to fold yourself into an extreme aero position then you would be well served to be genetically biased slightly towards the mobile end. As an aside, I remember a conversation with a Directeur Sportif at a Trek Factory Racing training camp in Calpe in 2013. He was concerned that their new protégé rider (Bob Jungels) had turned up at the camp with a hugely aggressive and potentially unsustainable riding position. When we put Jungels through an FMS it was clear he was both remarkably flexible and well-conditioned – he had that enviable ability to fold his long limbs into an impossibly contorted aero tuck and yet still function at 100 per cent of his power potential. This is what makes great champion cyclists – they support great genetics with specific conditioning work. Those of us who aren't so fortunate have to accept our genetic shortcomings and go heavy on the late-night homework – there are no shortcuts. At the time we had never measured a saddle-to-bar drop like the one Jungels had – I seem to remember it was 17 or even 19cm! But we reported back to the DS that his unique morphology and conditioning meant that his position was probably appropriate for him and sustainable, but also worth keeping a watch on as the season unfolded. Moreover, Jungels is a TT specialist and in our experience they like to set up their road bikes as close as they can to their TT bikes – maybe because they can?

The postscript to this story is that Jungels later came to us by himself and asked us to revise his position, to make it more comfortable and sustainable on long Grand Tour stages. In our opinion, that's the best way to work with any athlete or client – get them to be responsible for their own riding positions and let the issues and questions percolate down naturally over time. That way we're being used as collaborative consultants on their 'fit journey' (sorry). Some of the older riders in the team, who were closer to hanging up their wheels, just couldn't make this leap – they hadn't changed their bike set-up in 20 years and were not going to change now. They didn't understand that they didn't actually have to cede any control to us or, in fact, that it would have been wrong if they did.

If you go into a hairdresser and come out with a platinum perm or Mohican, just whose fault is it? OK, add great flexibility into our perfect theoretical cyclist – what's next?

Next up is ideal skeletal muscle make-up and physiology. We learned in chapter 1 that muscles are made up of a combination of slow- and fast-twitch fibre types. Fast-twitch fibres are the bigger and bulkier power muscles, ideal for explosive efforts and torque outputs. They have the ability to contract rapidly but also fatigue quicker as they aren't aerobically fuelled. Slow-twitch muscles fibres are superb at endurance and are aerobically fuelled by rich, oxygenated blood – hence they work best for torque and power outputs over a longer period of time. Most of our muscle groups are made up of both types, depending upon their specific task. For example, the muscles that control our eye movements are fast-twitch to allow quick, darting movements. But the postural muscles that control our trunk position tend to be slow-twitch, as they have to work all day long to control our orientation in relation to the ground (or office chair!). So what do we need for cycling? Well, that depends. If you're Sir Chris Hoy and you need to produce 2500 watts for a handful of seconds around a velodrome, then a matching set of 68.5cm thighs will come in very handy. But if you're Chris Froome, huge thighs add unnecessary bulk and weight because you'll spend your racing life with the dial hovering closer to 400 watts at the end of a mountain stage. While 400 watts is quite a handy output, it's still a fraction of what Froome would be capable of in an intense sprint burst and would be therefore mainly sustained by his oxygen-rich, slow-twitch muscle. Professional cyclists tend to have a ratio of around 80 per cent slow-twitch to 20 per cent fast-twitch muscles. The bunch sprinters will have a little more and the pure climbers a little less, but our theoretical perfect cyclist should have close to that 80–20 split.

The pelvis is king, the foot is prince, the knee is slave
Skeletally we would like our theoretically perfect cyclist to have a direct line of power from their anterior superior illiac spine (ASIS) through the

middle of the knee to their subtalar joint. Viewed from the front, think of a vertical line that bisects the front of your hip, through the knee and through the middle of your ankle. In cycling, the pelvis is held in place by the saddle and the foot is held by the pedal (aside from your ability to shift on the saddle and float slightly in the pedals). This kinetic chain is a victim of the positioning of the contact points. There are virtually no alignment choices that your body can make once the pedals are rotating and the chain is in motion. Any skeletal characteristic that affects the line from the ASIS (front of hip) to the subtalar joint potentially represents adverse loading and loss of function over time. That whole explanation could have been replaced by one sentence – performance cycling benefits from straight legs! An example of the kind of deviations from this perfect line of power is an issue such as tibial-varum, an inward curve of the tibia in the lower legs (or less politely, bow legs). Different hip architecture can also drive lower-limb conformation. Anteversion and retroversion describe the different positions of the femoral neck and the femoral shaft (the femur being the big bone in your upper leg). Too much retroversion will likely move the knee too far laterally (outward), which could increase loads through the knee and hip as you cycle. Too much anteversion can drive the knee too far medially (inside) and even send the foot pigeon-toed. Now think about your favourite cyclists and guess at their biomechanical predispositions. It's useful to return to a very old aphorism – and I can't remember where I first heard it: the pelvis is king, the foot is prince, the knee is slave. The knee is a victim of forces coming north from the hip and pelvis architecture, and south from the foot architecture and structure. If you see a professional rider with one or both knees flying out laterally at the top of the pedal stroke, consider if it's caused by:

1   Tibial-varum
2   Hip retroversion
3   Foot architecture and posture

4   Tightness in lateral structures around the hip – glute-meds, glutes, piriformis, etc.
5   Something else – more data needed

So welcome to our world. The answer is, of course, number five, something else; it's way too early to say. Look at an athlete like Peter Sagan, probably the best overall physical specimen in the pro peloton: why is he so pigeon-toed when he pedals, especially on the right foot? His excessive foot posture has, in my opinion, caused him to unclip in the sprint on at least one occasion. He's a devastatingly powerful athlete, but he's not a graceful pedaller – his biomechanics seem to be driving an exit strategy from the pedals on every stroke.

By the way, the most perfect cyclist we ever worked with was not a professional but an amateur called Warrick Spence, who worked as a bike fitter with us at Cyclefit for many years. Warrick raced and regularly won at elite level in the UK, even without a team. He didn't train as much as his fellow (mostly professional) racers because he worked full time. We tested his VO$_2$ max at 82 in the off-season, so he had a huge engine, but don't they all at that level? What set Warrick apart was an innate conformation and grace on his bicycle – his body worked best in that medium for all the reasons I have highlighted above. He was symmetrical and flexible, and also had flawless muscle morphology and perfect lower-limb skeletal alignment and foot architecture. Warrick looked like a climber in terms of his appearance but regularly won bunch sprints, and while he couldn't push 2500 watts like Chris Hoy, he could drive long enough at 850 watts to wear everybody down in the last kilometre. Warrick was (and still is) a one-man squad, who never seemed to get injured or suffer pain. To his fellow racers he was an anomaly – kooky and kind-hearted off the bike, but almost unassailable on it – but they never knew why. We did: he was born to be a bike rider, one of those extraordinary humans who have evolved to ride bikes, a rare exception that proves our rule.

The cycling body: the curious incidence of time and events

Even the Warricks of this world aren't immune to either time or events. Both have an inevitable consequence on how the rider relates to their bike and the athletic act of cycling. The difference between cycling and running is that the inevitable adaptations and compensations with the former tend to happen under our conscious radar, whereas with running these changes are more obvious. To illustrate, let's say that you strain a hamstring playing rounders in a charity tournament for your daughter's school (in no way a real example). Should you try to run the next day, the pain and loss of function will be acute and obvious – it will hurt a great deal and you will limp. Switch immediately to the bike, and the pain may well be completely dialled down in that moment, but that may be due to the body adapting around the tightness. This could make the foot more plantarflexed (toe-down) on the injured side to control (lessen) the knee-extension angle. This may in turn increase joint loading forces on the front of the knee or make the pelvis unstable (depending on hip-in-flexion range). In addition, the uninjured side may start trying to help (again unconsciously) and start pulling up on the pedals (almost always a bad idea) and overwork the hip flexors. The body will also make adaptions for running and walking, but the central distinction is that you'll probably be aware of them and what they mean. Try to run with an acute hamstring strain, and it will hurt, and you'll stop. Try to cycle, and it may hurt considerably less, but that does not mean that unhelpful adaptations aren't taking place.

Sometimes the events are more severe than a hamstring strain at a rounders game, which you haven't played for at least 35 years and for which you did absolutely no warm-up or stretching. It's safe to assume that Eddy Merckx possessed one of the finest cycling physiques ever to wander our planet on a bicycle. He was almost certainly a 'Burtian' macro-absorber and also a 'Fugallo-optimum' specimen in terms of strength-to-flexibility ratio. Merckx was also arguably the greatest all-rounder of any sport in history – his competitors were never safe – and he could sprint, climb and time trial better than most of the specialists. He was the Muhammad Ali of cycling – fast, ruthless and powerful. In 1969 he was 24 years old and enjoying a superb season – victories in the Tour of Flanders and Milan–San Remo, and domination of the 56th Tour de France. The kind of season that makes the Grand Tour winners of the recent era look a little bland and cossetted.

On 9 September, Merckx participated in a three-stage omnium track event in Blois, France. During the first stage, Merckx and Fernand Wambst, his derny driver (a derny is a small motorbike used to pace the cyclist), were involved in a serious accident with another derny and competitor. Wambst died in the crash and Merckx was seriously injured and rendered unconscious by the trackside. He spent a week in hospital with injuries to his back, pelvis and head. From that point forward Merckx permanently pivoted, I believe, from a supple macro-absorber into a hyper-tense micro-adjuster. The monstrous engine pretty much returned, seemingly undimmed, to full horsepower, but the chassis was always fragile from that moment to the end of his career. One can only imagine how many Grand Tours and one-day races Merckx would have won without that crash, and it may be one reason why he's now famously reluctant to talk about his racing past. I remember trying to coax him a few times to talk about the old days and he was totally intractable on the matter. The most I would get was 'The past is the past is the past – I just wish I could go back and do it all better.'

There's a prescient scene in Jorgen Leth's spellbinding film *A Sunday In Hell*, about the 1976 running of the Paris–Roubaix race. The whole Molteni squad is seen riding en masse to the start of the race, with Merckx the senior patron, an already fading grand champion, continually stopping and fiddling with his bike, even stopping the team car and reaching in for a wrench to make another futile adjustment. It was an endless process of frustrating biomechanical discombobulation around a strained physiology that was endlessly adapting around poor positioning. He was trying to hit a permanently shifting bullseye wearing a blindfold – it was an impossible task. I'm sure that if we could travel back in time, with all the knowledge, diagnostic tools and technology that we have now, it would be possible to make his situation substantially better – orthotics, shorter cranks, more suitable pelvic support and so on may even have prolonged his stellar career for a few more seasons. But it would all be based on the post-1969, new normal that he woke up with after the crash at Blois. To a career bike fitter, the Paris–Roubaix film scene is just heartbreaking – all we want to do is lead him away from the impending suffering of the world's most brutal bike race into our quiet fitting studio to run a few hours' worth of diagnostics and adjustments to make things more tolerable for him. He lost the 1976 Paris–Roubaix race to Marc Demeyer by the way, after a typically heroic and stoic performance.

In truth we're all a permanently moving bullseye due to incremental attritions in age, health, fitness, injury, stress and weight. Generally the increments are small and imperceptible and can be reviewed just once or twice per year. The Merckx accident of '69 was a life deflection that could neither be undone or recalibrated for at that time. It was always simply a question of how much pain Merckx could endure through his physical fuselage as he progressed through his career. He retired in 1978 at the age of 33 with 525 victories on his palmares – that's quite enough pain for anyone.

Not a robot – age-related cycling biomechanical issues

A question we often hear in the Cyclefit studios goes something like: 'I have done 100,000km in this position and then all of a sudden my foot/knee/hip/neck/pelvis is agony – what is going on?'

You're not a robot is what's going on and, even if you were, robots break down eventually. Just as you could spend your whole life in your theoretically perfect cycling biomechanical place, there would probably still be deterioration through repetition. It's just inevitable – it's plainly impossible to reduce every friction, micro-trauma and tension in your body as you fight the effects of ageing. Our bodies are remarkable and as we get older, and no longer have youth on our side, we would be well advised to appreciate them more. Newly qualified doctors and clinicians often can't wait to intervene to fix an illness or an injury – they are filled with a 'zeal to heal'. More experienced clinicians long ago learned that our bodies will heal themselves and will do most of the heavy lifting connected with healing and renewal – the clinicians' most important role, therefore, is to support the environment that will allow restoration and renewal to take place. Doctors don't generate new bone when you have a fracture – osteogenesis happens quite naturally within your own body. It's the medic's role to support the process by making sure that the bones are properly aligned and supported throughout this natural healing process. Most of modern medicine, physical therapy and, to a certain degree, bike fitting is predicated on this process.

The primary difference with bike fitting is when the bike or bike position is actually driving the pain or injury – that's to say, the pain isn't provoked by any other activity. At that point the experienced bike fitter becomes a detective looking for the underlying cause – what is it about the way this person is interacting with this bicycle and all of its contact points and components which is adversely directing their body? Our mission is to offload the structures that are painful or injured, while at the same time maintaining the athlete's full function. Sometimes that's not possible, or not possible immediately. On many occasions, clients have limped into the studio, maybe a few days away from a big event, filled with anxiety because they're in so much pain and they fear a whole season's training will be wasted if they can't participate. On most occasions it's already far too late to help sufficiently to enable them to compete. There's simply no point in raising expectations or making their situation worse. Our job is to be professional and refer them to the right clinician or therapist for a clinical diagnosis or treatment. This is rarely what they want to hear, and some assume that deep in our bike fit studios we have some magic fairy dust we can sprinkle in such emergencies. Sadly not – modern bike studios should be places filled with pragmatism and practicality, rooted in what's possible and what's absolutely not. The two most powerful tools we have at our disposal are the ability to say the words 'I don't know' and 'no', and not dive down imaginary rabbit holes, probably making things worse by offering false promises. If a client walks in with a suspected herniated disc, the proper place for them is the waiting room in a doctor's surgery, A&E or therapist – maybe all three.

Although we have no access to magic fairy dust, we can often help injured riders in very sensible ways. Here are the most common injuries and niggles that we see every day, how ageing contributes, and what we do to try and help.

Foot pain

More people present, or are referred, with foot pain than any other issue; it's our number one problem to fix. Cycling foot pain is quite unlike other kinds of pain because there's no possible relief unless you stop and take your shoes off. If your bottom hurts you can stand up off the saddle; if your back hurts you can extend or flex to try and get a moment's relief; too much pressure on your hands and you can take them off the bars and shake them around. None of that's possible with your feet – their position is predetermined by the relationship with the shoe, cleat, pedal and crank.

Remember, bipeds are actually very rare in nature – kangaroos, ostriches and some primates (who only have the capacity to be bipedal on occasions) pretty much make up the whole list. Consequently our feet have evolved to be remarkable, complex structures made up of 33 joints, 28 bones, 107 ligaments and 19 muscle/tendon attachments. An unbelievable quarter of all your bones are in your feet.

Being bipedal means that our feet have a huge amount of work to do to exert power and control in relation to the ground. In terms of the function of the foot, it's important to understand that running and walking are entirely opposite to cycling. Cyclefit podiatrist Mick Habgood says: 'In relation to foot function – walking and running are all about facilitating movement and in cycling it's all about blocking movement.'

The movement we're trying to 'block' in cycling is in the 'sagittal plane' – looking down at your feet from above, the movement from the little toe towards the big toe (or the other way). Look down on your feet, and you will see how much bigger the first MPJ (big-toe joint) is than the others. The sooner we can get connection through the first MPJ, then the earlier power will be developed through the foot into the pedal. Hence, we want to block the side-to-side rocking movement to facilitate early power connection. The degree to which the foot pivots around its long axis when you pedal is contingent on your foot type. Mick Habgood again: 'The feet you have today are a product of what you were born with and what you have done to them over time – footwear, lifestyle, sport and trauma.'

Your feet will necessarily change over time as you age. You may not have had a bunion when you were born but you're born with the mechanics and predisposition to get one in later life. These changes happen over decades of mechanical loading. The important thing to remember is that your feet are changing over time, and these changes could cause issues at the foot, knee, hip, back or even higher up.

Pain across the metatarsals (ball of the foot)

This is very common and incredibly difficult to endure on longer rides, especially if it's hot – in fact, it's sometimes referred to as 'hot foot'. If the pain or numbness extends across the metatarsals it could be that the shoe is too narrow, which is compressing the nerves between the metatarsals, resulting in pain or numbness. Lateral pain across the metatarsals can also be caused by incorrect cleat position or pedal choice. Twenty years ago we used to place the centre of the pedal spindle right over the second metatarsal – further forward than the first metatarsal. The theory was that the foot is a first-class lever, where the ankle is the pivot, the ground (pedal) is the load and the calf muscles represent the force – a perfect see-saw. Pushing the cleat forward over the second metatarsal made the foot lever longer and therefore provided greater mechanical advantage. And so it probably did, but it was also unsustainable for many folk because it increased irritation through the plantar nerves between the metatarsals. Now we start with the middle of the cleat positioned 8–12mm behind the first metatarsal.

Fifth metatarsal pain

Fifth metatarsal pain is high up in our all-time top 10 and can be caused simply by an inappropriate shoe, meaning the last is too narrow or the wrong design or shape for your foot. For example, some shoes curve inwards in a slight banana shape from the heel to the toe. But if your foot naturally moves in the opposite direction, then pressure could be felt on the outside of the foot. The other cause of lateral pressure could be foot posture – you may have a foot with forefoot supinatus (the big toe is tilted up towards the midline), which could load the fifth metatarsal. The remedies here could be a footbed or orthotic and possible medial wedging inside or outside of the shoe. Alternatively you may have a pes cavus foot (high arch) that tends to load up the outside edge the foot/shoe. There's one other possible cause – stance width. If the cleat–pedal position is set up too narrow, the athlete may feel pressure down the lateral column (outside), which may extend into the side of the knee and hip. This is potentially a very easy self-help fix – move the cleat in and the foot out. Sometimes it's necessary to step the foot even further out, to protect an externally rotating knee. This can be achieved using Shimano SPDSL +4mm pedals or, if you need more (and plenty of people do), Speedplay pedals with changeable axle widths.

We've a saying at Cyclefit, 'fit the foot first', meaning that optimising the foot–pedal interface is the most important aspect of your bike connection. It's no wonder professional cyclists are fastidious to the point of obsession about their shoe–cleat–pedal set-up, and they dread the day that they have to change shoe or pedal sponsors.

I remember very well working with a World Tour team, with Jules, at their training camp in Spain at the end of the year – they were changing both shoe and pedal sponsor at the same time. The mood of the camp was tense as riders would come back off their morning training spins and ride their bikes straight into our fitting areas, desperate to download their unredacted feedback to the assembled fit crew, even before having a shower and lunch! And we, in turn, were very keen to hear what they had to say – particularly because changing shoes and pedals had changed all of their internal knee-extension angles (the stack height of the shoe and pedal was different from the shoe and pedal they were moving from). Most let us change their saddle height to compensate, but some didn't. It was the latter group that we wanted to monitor in case they experienced compensations elsewhere – for example in the foot, Achilles, knee, hip and back. Generally, all the feedback was initially negative (pro riders, for good reason, dislike change), as the sensations were all unfamiliar and therefore unwelcome. Their instinct was to try to control the unfamiliar by blocking the movement at the pedal interface by taking away all of the float – almost always a bad idea. Our job was to suggest a reflection of their normal walking mechanics in their cycling foot posture. But ultimately it's their decision – we're purely sounding boards. But before you set your own pedals up with zero float, have someone film you in slow motion from the front as you walk towards them. Look at the phase of motion that the foot goes through and imagine how that would feel if this movement was prevented. Blocking internal/external rotation can drive a compensation movement up into the knee and/or hip. It's important to remember that internal/external rotation (foot moving heel-in or heel-out as we pedal) is different to the rocking motion – in general, we want to reflect and facilitate the former and lock down the latter

I should point out that we don't clip into pedals in cycling shoes in order to pull up – we clip in to keep the foot stable and in the most functional and comfortable position on the pedal. (We discuss this much more when we look at the pedal stroke later in this chapter.)

Achilles tendonitis

Achilles issues are more common with running and sports with ballistic movements – the classic injury occurs in the jump and reach when serving in tennis, causing a rupture or tear. Less serious injuries are less acute and more chronic and build up over time. We learned in chapter 1 that as we get older the collagen fibre matrix can become a little more disorganised and therefore prone to injury. The big problem with Achilles issues is that they have an annoying tendency to rumble on, and it can therefore be difficult to treat. Physical therapists will assess the degree of damage and set up a rehab programme to de-stress the structure and then try to build future resilience through strength and conditioning. Treating Achilles issues on the bike is predicated on two strategies – one, find the underlying cause and two, offload the Achilles structure. In terms of the first, it's not always possible, because even if the athlete rides two hours every day, that still leaves a possible 22 hours doing other things that may be stressing the tendon. Possible underlying causes and potential fixes on the bike are:

- Foot stability. Pronation or supination (the action of the foot rotating around its long axis) can adversely load the Achilles structure. Fix: Support the foot with an orthotic or footbeds and stabilise the foot on the pedal with internal (inside the shoe) and/or external (under the cleat) wedges.

- Calf weakness. This can result in an inability to maintain a plantar-flexed (toes-down) foot attitude in the pedal stroke, or excessive dorsiflexion (toes-up). Fix: Physical therapist-led plan to increase calf strength and appropriate range of motion.

- Poor bike positioning. This is generally a result of the saddle being too far back and/or too high. Fix: Lower the saddle and/or re-set fore/aft saddle position.

- Asymmetry. An anatomically (due to bone length) or functionally (due to compensation) shorter leg can cause tightness and Achilles issues over time. Fix: Possible leg-length compensation with a stack and/or physical therapy to correct a functional asymmetry.

- Muscle tightness. A shortness or tightness in calves or hamstrings can provoke Achilles issues. Fix: Stretching and or physical therapy. Alex Fugallo suggests starting with a one-legged neutral heel stance (toes on a step and stand suspended with the heel and toes at the same height), which he calls 'paracetamol for Achilles tendons', before going on to do heel-drop and calf strengthening exercises.

- Incorrect cleat position, shoe or pedal. All can contribute to Achilles issues building up over time. Fix: Shorten the foot lever by bringing the cleats all the way back to offload the Achilles and calf. This can be temporary or permanent.

- Poor pedalling technique. This can negatively affect loading through the Achilles – for example, using high torque and low cadences when climbing can cause excessive heel drop and adverse forces at the tendon. Fix: Retrain the pedalling technique (see more later in this chapter).

The knee

As we've seen, the knee is susceptible to forces moving south from the hip/pelvis and also moving north from the foot. The knee joint is the biggest in the body and is described as a 'modified hinge joint', which means that it facilitates predominantly flexion and extension (straightening and bending of the leg) but also a limited degree of internal and external rotation. So what can go wrong with a cyclist's knee over time, with an accumulation of traumatic events, and combined forces from the foot and the hip?

Anterior knee pain

The biggest issue we see is simple patellofemoral pain, or anterior knee pain (AKP). This occurs at the front of the knee, generally caused by compression forces acting on the knee cap (patella) via the patella tendon. The fixes can be a simple repositioning of the saddle, normally increasing the internal knee-extension angle, but can also be more complex, involving muscle-recruitment balances. Typically, an over-reliance on knee-extensor muscles (quadriceps) over glutes (hip-extensor muscles) is the result of poor posture, positioning on the bike or poor technique. Some riders neglect to use their powerful glutes, leaving their quad (thigh) muscles a huge amount of work to do. Sometimes we want to reduce the compressive forces on the front of the patella to reduce pain by increasing the knee-extension angle. The easy fix is to increase saddle height, but we can't because there's a tightness or shortness in the posterior chain (hamstring and calves). This posterior tightness introduces a frictional tug-of-war into the dynamic chain between the knee extensors (quadriceps) and knee flexors (hamstrings and calves). The net outcome is that we push the saddle up to increase the knee internal angle and the athlete unconsciously compensates by plantar-flexing the foot more than usual (positioning the toes down) to reduce the knee angle to offload their posterior chain. The only practical solution at this point is a stretching regime to increase tolerance of an increased knee angle.

Medial knee pain

The second-highest incidence of problems is cyclists presenting with medial knee pain (pain on the inside of the knee). By definition, this will be a rotational torque control issue rather than one arising from compressive forces. This rotational influence could be coming down from the hip in terms of glute control or up from the foot. Leaving aside the hip/pelvis element, because this would fall more to a physical therapist or a strength and conditioning coach, the foot forces that we seek to optimise fall into two movement planes:

1 Pronation – movement in the sagittal plane (rocking), caused by foot posture. Fix: Orthotics or cycling footbed, medial wedging (would be built into cycling orthotic).

2 Rotation/stance – internal/external rotation of the foot in the pedal. Fix: Optimise the pedal float profile and cleat rotation with neutral foot position. Locking the foot outside of the neutral foot position could force a release to the joint above – the knee. The general rule is that if you walk like a duck (toes out), then that's how your cleats should be set up. If you walk like a pigeon (toes in), your cleats should be set up to accommodate that. Over the years, we've had amateur and professional cyclists observe that they have excessive rotation at the foot and have sought to control this natural movement at the cleat–pedal interface, which frequently has painful consequences. As we get older, our tolerances for these misalignments tends to decrease. I can't think of circumstances (outside of the track) where I would recommend a midlife athlete pedal without any float at all in their pedal set-up.

It's also worth pointing out that stance width could also have a deleterious effect on both medial and lateral knee pain. Medial knee pain is incredibly common but also, generally speaking, one of the easier issues to correct through good bike fitting practices.

An added complication that's worth mentioning is tibial torsion, which is a twist in the shin bone (tibia) below the knee. A tibial torsion will either internally or externally push the foot out of line with the knee (the foot points either toes in or toes out). Not all foot rotations are caused by tibial torsions, but all tibial torsions will cause foot rotations. It's vital that the foot rotation is adequately reflected in the foot position on the pedal or persistent knee pain can occur. If you run with a tibial torsion, the foot will automatically find its own pathway, but in cycling it's perfectly possible to effectively trap the foot in a poor position.

Iliotibial band syndrome (ITBS)

This is another very common biomechanical problem for both cyclists and triathletes. Thankfully, it has a mostly straightforward and rational fix. ITBS is normally felt on the outside of the knee, where the iliotibial band (ITB) creates a friction inflammation as it passes over the bony landmark called the lateral femoral epicondyle (bony landmark on the outside of the knee). The ITB is a fascia structure (a thin sheath of connective tissue) with the tensile strength of steel, which runs down the lateral side (outside) of the leg. At the top of the leg, the ITB runs into the tensor fascia latae (TFL) muscle. Together the ITB and TFL are lateral rotators or abductors (which move the leg outwards), as well as being knee stabilisers. ITB pain is particularly gruelling and very challenging to ignore – clients report being brought to a virtual standstill by ITBS, when the pain can become hot and stabbing in nature. ITBS shouldn't be underestimated because it can easily become chronic and harder to resolve, even when the underlying causes have been corrected (it's a bit like Achilles tendonitis in this regard). Possible potential ITBS causes and fixes could be:

- Stance width. Setting feet too close together will increase the incidence of friction at the side of the knee. Fix: Increase stance width by moving cleats inwards or using wider pedal spindles, such as those found on Shimano SPSL or Speedplay pedals.
- Pronation at the foot. This can increase ITBS. Fix: Use orthotics and medial wedges.
- Saddle height. Setting the saddle too high can increase ITB friction. Fix: Lower the saddle.
- Poor glute or hip control. This can overwork the TFL and ITB. Fix: Specific strength and conditioning work, as well as using a shorter crank.
- Poor hip-in-flexion range. This can prompt femur, and therefore knee, abduction (movement outwards), which will increase pressure on the lateral (outside) structures and create sensitivity or pain. Fix: Increase the hip range, reduce crank length and increase stance width.

Medial plica syndrome

To be clear: this is not a common problem, but it is out there, and we do see it occasionally. I mention it because it is intrinsically difficult to diagnose without an MRI scan and a consultant like Dr Hulse (who also used to be a knee surgeon in a previous life). Medial plica syndrome is often diagnosed by exclusion, meaning that we refer clients to Dr Hulse when no other fixes work. The knee is a synovial joint, which means that the upper and lower leg bones are surrounded by a fibrous capsule that's filled with viscous liquid called synovial fluid. A plica is a tiny wrinkle in the synovial capsule, thought to be a leftover from our time developing in the womb. When the athlete pedals, the plicae can tug or catch on surrounding structures and cause pain and inflammation. There's no specific bike-fit fix; anything we try has to be physician-led. It should also be said that every athlete we've worked with who has had keyhole (arthroscopic) surgery for this issue has returned to full-time training and racing. Start thinking medial plica syndrome (other plicae can be affected, but they are rarer in our experience) if you've persistent knee pain when you ride and no other remedies have relieved the symptoms.

The hips

Like the knee, the hip joint is a synovial joint, meaning it's surrounded by a fibrous capsule and filled with super-lubricated synovial fluid. The hip joint refers to the ball on the end of the thigh bone (femur) where it meets the socket (acetabulum) located on the pelvis. Unlike the knee, which is a hinge joint, the hip joint is a ball and socket joint and therefore has a greater range of motion – it comprises (ideally) rotational movement as well as extension and flexion of the hip. It's our opinion that the construction of the hip and pelvis (the architecture of the neck of the femur and acetabulum) is one of the fundamental predicates that separates good from great cyclists, and their ability to train and race tens of thousands of kilometres per year. Why? Because the hip is the primary connection between your lower limb skeleton, where all the power is produced and transmitted, and the 80 bones of your axial skeleton (spine/skull etc), which forms an essential stabilisation and control function. The hip and pelvis is, in effect, your bottom bracket. The hip is also an area that seems to be especially vulnerable to both trauma and age-related degeneration. If you fall off your bike, the large bump you can feel on the outside of your hip (the greater trochanter) is especially exposed and can transmit injuries to the thigh bone, hip joint and pelvis. We're usually always working with at least one athlete who is recovering from a trauma to the hip area.

The hip joint is also especially prone to degeneration from ageing – another reason to avoid becoming osteopenic or osteoporotic as we get older (see chapter 1). In fact, many clients have reported finding out that they were suffering from hip bone degeneration only as a result of a DEXA scan post-crash. This provokes the inevitable question as to whether the crash injury was exacerbated because of osteopenia or osteoporosis.

Bike-related hip issues

As we've seen, hip-in-flexion range is the ability to bring the femur close to the spine without bony or soft-tissue restriction. This range of motion is essential for resilience to cycling intensity and duration. It's also unique to cycling because riding a bike demands that you function at a high level with a closed hip and flexed spine. We already mentioned that for a professional female cyclist we like to see around 130 degrees of hip-in-flexion range. For a professional male this should be around 120 degrees. For amateur women and men, anything above 110 degrees is good. Below 100 degrees, and it becomes necessary to make significant changes to the bike set-up to prevent a loss of comfort and function. By the way, after hip replacement surgery, patients are frequently directed to avoid moving the hip into flexion beyond 90 degrees, at least during the rehab period. Remember, cycling is highly prescriptive – you cannot choose the range of motion your hip is operating at during the pedalling cycle. The range of motion is being minutely directed by a combination of crank length, saddle height and position, ankling-patterning (dorsiflexion or plantar flexion) and pelvis and spine posture. A hip-in-flexion restriction can result in the hip and knee abducting (moving outward) around the restriction, which in turn can cause hip, knee and foot pain, and a loss of power. A hip restriction can also result in a loss of stability on the saddle, which can cause pain or even saddle sores. And finally a lack of hip range can result in pain into the lower, mid or even upper parts of the back as a compensation. If the range issue is caused by a bony impediment such as a bone spur or a degeneration of the hip, the underlying cause must be assessed by a doctor. You may be able to continue to ride but you'll need to make changes to your bike set-up, to open up the hip angle. Try these fixes:

1　Shorten your crank
2　Raise your handlebars
3　Reduce your saddle setback behind the bottom bracket (to further open the hip)
4　Raise your saddle as far as hamstring/calf tightness will allow (within upper range)

If the impediment is soft tissue – tightness in the muscles around the hip (glutes, glute-meds, piriformis, hip-flexors, hamstrings, almost everything) – you would be well advised to start a targeted stretching and conditioning routine to increase the hip-in-flexion range. This will revolutionise your pedal stroke (excuse the pun).

Hip flexors

I don't want to stray too far into hip flexors because we cover the topic in some detail below (see p. 194). But clients do come to us with tightness in their hip flexors, almost always accompanied by some degree of pedal stroke dysfunction and maybe poor rehab from injury. 'Hip flexor' is arguably a misdirecting term that encompasses a motley selection of muscles which have quantitatively disparate effects on the action of hip flexion. The rectus femoris, for example, is a member of your quadricep group at the front of your thigh. It's a knee extender, along with all your quads, but because it crosses the hip, it's also a hip extender. The 'rec fem' (as it's called) can be a troubling little muscle for cyclists if it tightens up under load. And then there's the 'strongest' of the hip flexor group, the iliopsoas, comprising the illiacus (which attaches to the iliac fossa (the internal smooth surface of the pelvis) and the psoas major (which attaches to your lower lumbar vertebrae). The bike fitter's role here is to chase down the underlying cause – stretching may give short-term relief and range but will not help in the longer term unless we find out what is actually traumatising the muscle structures. Generally speaking, pain in the front of the hip – which may also be felt in the lumbar area (where the psoas is attached) – is caused by an inappropriate reliance on these structures during cycling. They are relatively weak and, in the case of the psoas group, are also muscles that we rely on to stabilise our trunk position, meaning they are are postural. Here are some possible hip flexor bike fit fixes:

1 Stop clipping in, for a while at least, and use flat pedals instead (see 'The perfect pedal stroke' below, p. 194).
2 Raise your handlebars, so that the hip flexors don't have to perform their trunk stabilising job.
3 Shorten your cranks, to reduce compression into the hip area at the top of the pedal stroke.
4 Improve your seated posture by avoiding slouching.
5 Check your saddle position (fore/aft and height), but also your choice of saddle design.

Our general rule (and this is probably contentious) is that hip flexors have a role in cycling as trunk stabilisers and to influence pelvic and spinal posture, but should have a very minimal (read zero) part in actual power production – i.e. do not pull up on the pedals. Nothing good ever comes from the hip flexors in cycling!

The pelvis

The foot may be the most common cause of pain in cycling overall, but for women, saddle- or pelvis-related pain is the number one issue that they would like resolved. Someone (who should know) told us a frightening statistic recently – 90 per cent of professional female riders have saddle-related issues at some point in their career. Our own experience working with athletes at every level, from recreational through to professional, validates that. To be clear: nine out of ten female cyclists that we work with have, or have had, saddle-related pain or problems. That's a pretty sad indictment of the cycling industry, which has manifestly failed to properly support, literally and metaphorically, women in the sport. By contrast, over the 20 years we've been working with clients in the bike fit studio, saddle pain affects around 33 per cent of men.

Having said that, humans didn't really evolve to sit down at all – chairs were invented only around 5000 years ago – never mind sit down and produce maximum power. This is all the fault of the Victorians, of course (not that we've done much to correct their errors). Dr Tim Briggs, consultant urological surgeon and high-level midlife cyclist, lists these factors as contributing to the high incidence of saddle pressure pain and associated medical issues:

- Aged over 50 – the incidence of saddle pain increases with age.
- Higher body weight – more weight equals more pressure on the saddle.
- Over 10 years of cycling and training – physical issues seem to be cumulative.
- Intensity of training – more than three hours of cycling per week.

As midlife athletes, we seem to tick quite a few of Dr Brigg's high-risk boxes – but what are the underlying causes and what can we do about it?

The pudendal canal and pudendal nerve entrapment syndrome

So why are high-output efforts while seated on a minimal saddle a problem? Dr Briggs says: 'Pedalling while sitting on a slim, hard saddle and being subject to repetitive impacts generates extreme perineal pressure which indirectly compresses the pudendal nerves and increases the friction within the pudendal canal.'

This doesn't sound great, does it? The pudendal nerve is the key nerve of the pelvic floor and perineum. The pudendal arteries share scarce real estate with the pudendal nerve as they both travel within the pudendal canal. Compression of these structures can cause pain, numbness and permanent damage if ignored over time. Dr Briggs thinks that this pressure is exacerbated by the simple action of pedalling: 'The movements of the pedalling legs in the forward sitting position stretch the pudendal nerves over the 'sacro spinous' and 'sacro tuberous' ligaments.' Here are some possible pudendal canal pressure solutions:

1. Change your saddle. Don't buy a saddle on looks alone; go through a diagnostic procedure to find one that suits your individual pelvic architecture. Point of interest: Dr Briggs was actually using a saddle that was significantly too wide for his narrow sit-bones, which meant that he slid forwards on the saddle to find a narrower section. This made him unstable and also affected his knee extension angle. Make sure you always stand up and pedal periodically. We consider a mix of standing and sitting to be a superior pedalling technique (see 'The perfect pedal stroke' below, p. 194).

2. Review your cycling posture and bike fit to make sure that you're positioned properly on the saddle and maximising your glute contraction. Well-developed and engaged glutes will offload sensitive soft-tissue.

3. There is no such thing as 'breaking in a new saddle' – a saddle either works for your pelvis construction or it doesn't.

4. Never set your saddle nose-up. We recommend 0 to -2 degrees of nose-down for men, and 0 to -4 degrees for women.

Vulval lymphoedema

This is saddle-related and is the result of excessive pressure on female soft tissue. It's incredibly common and can be painful and distressing. And sometimes it's been impossible for us to find a satisfactory long-term solution in the context of the fitting studio, even when we've applied pressure-mapping technology across an almost infinite supply of female-specific saddles. I would go as far as to say that this is the area of our greatest collective professional exasperation. But the situation is improving all the time as more research is undertaken, and better products subsequently emerge. Here's what we suggest as possible fixes:

- Review your bike fit – for example, a saddle set too high will dramatically increase soft tissue pressure.
- Set your saddle between 0–4 degrees nose-down, but no more or you'll load up your arms and shoulders too much.
- Shorten your cranks to reduce pedalling circumference and increase stability.
- Try an alternative design, such as an ISM or other 'nose-less' saddle.
- Get into the habit of standing more, especially when you climb. Climbing will make the nose more positively slanted, which we want to avoid.
- Maintain core function so you are intrinsically stable on the saddle.
- Don't run your handlebars too far below your saddle if you have frontal saddle pressure – you can always go to the drops or put more of a bend in your elbow for situations where you need to go lower.
- Pain is about stability as well as outright pressure. Sometimes we see high pressure points that are well-tolerated and low pressures that are not – the missing piece is generally 'stability'. Instability

plus pressure equals pain. Change your position and posture on the bike and, if necessary, do some strength and conditioning to become more stable on the saddle.

- Fit the foot first. Something felt at the pelvis is often driven up from the foot. Issues include asymmetry, pronation and stability.

- Make sure you have the best cycling shorts you can afford – a bib short will keep the pad in the correct place and help offload pressure while you ride.

Saddle sores

It would be naïve to think I could write a book about cycling without mentioning boils on our nether regions. If you've ever had to endure one of these festering manifestations, you'll know it can wreck an event, a trip or even entire season.

Saddle sores share the same causes as vulval lymphoedema, in the sense that both are the result of localised loading and forces. We hear the same story from amateur and professional cyclists alike: 'I always get a saddle sore in exactly the same place.' Of course we do. Sores are not caused by a vengeful god (although that's often how they feel), they are an inevitable consequence of our changing biomechanics and their relationship to our contact points. The causative mechanism of saddle sores is a combination of pure pressure and sheer stress, caused by a lack of pelvis and saddle stability. But what is driving the excess pressure or lack of stability? And what can we do about it? Here are some issues and potential fixes:

- Incorrect saddle choice. It's a myth that big riders should have big saddles – incorrect saddle choice will mean inappropriate soft tissue and skeletal loading. The biggest riders can have the narrowest pelvises, and vice versa. You won't know until you go through a diagnostic procedure like pressure-mapping to find out.

If you use a saddle that's too narrow you may find that you shift your weight backwards, looking for a wider part of the saddle that doesn't exist. Use a saddle that's too wide and you may, unconsciously, scoot forwards to a narrower part that you prefer. The problem is this may change your centre of gravity and you may now be loading up your hands or closing your knee angle, or both. Fix: Find the right saddle for you, right now. Remember that your choice may need to change as you change, or a newer saddle becomes available.

- Poor bike fit. This will result in asymmetric stresses on your body, which will tip over into the contact point between the pelvis and saddle. After the feet, the pelvis is the next most crucial contact point. If you're tighter or shorter on the left-hand side of your body, it won't be remarkable that you get more pressure on that side. Over time a lesion or sore could form. Fix: Know your body and make sure your position reflects everything about it. For example, if you have had an ACL reconstruction made from your own hamstring, you may still have residual tightness on the side from where the tissue was harvested. This tightness could pull the pelvis down on one side and increase saddle pressure. You could try to lengthen the hamstring with stretching and conditioning, or compensate for the shortness with a small stack for a while – most likely both.

- Poor trunk and core strength. These could make you less stable on the saddle. Remember the rule – instability plus pressure equals pain. Fix: Great cyclists have great overall physical conditioning, of which trunk and core strength are their most treasured components.

- Poor technique and posture. Both could result in adverse loading onto the saddle. Slouching will tend to load up the sit bones (ischial tuberosities) and rotating too far forward could load up the pubic symphasis (a fibro-cartilage joint at the front of the pelvis). Going back to Alex Fugallo's hypermobile v stiff spectrum, very tight riders tend to be rotated backwards because of posterior chain tightness. By contrast, hypermobile riders may rotate forwards onto their pubic symphasis, looking for stability at the end of their range. Perhaps that may ring a few bells for some folk who are wondering why they are suffering from extreme loading patterns? Fix: Go back to the first principles of pedalling and sitting on a bike – a neutral spine (see 'The perfect pedal stroke' below, p. 194).

- Spending money on expensive chamois creams and shorts. By themselves, these purchases will not alleviate pressure sores – especially if the sores are asymmetric and regular. You must look for an underlying biomechanical cause.

Back pain

Cycling and back pain are almost as synonymous as cycling and saddle pain – clients often remark, 'Sure, my back hurts, but doesn't everyone's when they cycle?' The answer is no. And certainly not all of the time. The biggest bike-related contributor to back pain, beyond bike fit or an injury such as a herniated disc, is poor posture and technique. It's something we unconsciously do to ourselves.

First principles: we've evolved to be powerful in extension. Think of any power sport and the stance that will be adopted is the pelvis rotated forwards into neutral and the spine in extension. A sprinter exploding out of the blocks, the forwards locking into a scrum, a player waiting to return a service in tennis, a diver launching themselves into a pool all do it; even canoeists and rowers maximise power by lengthening through their spine at the vital catch with the water. The only outlier is cycling and the ability to rotate back (slouch) on the saddle and to flex the lumbar spine. The problem with this posture is that we evolved to produce maximum power with optimal protection for our spine. Rotating back, or slouching, is a passive posture, and inhibits co-contraction of our explosive glute muscles and essential trunk and core muscles. Co-contraction of the glutes and our trunk (core) muscles is key to our powerful function. We have evolved to have a dynamic and responsive relationship between the incredibly powerful glute muscle and the recruitment of the stabilising trunk group of muscles. This dynamic relationship delivers optimal power production and protection to the lower spine. Some riders rotate back because they unconsciously feel too much weight on their hands and slouching back is one method of unloading this pressure on the front of the bike. Other riders are pulled back into a passive position because they are too tight in the posterior chain. Some of us just do it because we can – it's a habit (my hand is up as I type, by the way).

Poor posture on the bike also negatively affects the whole length of the spine, including neck and head posture, often resulting in overworked upper trapezius muscles (which radiate from the side of the neck out to the shoulder) as we hyper-extend our head and neck so we can see down the road from our slouched stance. Female cyclists frequently cause neck or back pain by unconsciously rolling their pelvis backwards, away from uncomfortable frontal saddle pressure. The biomechanical consequences can be profound:

- Lack of trunk/core/back muscle contraction, which leaves the back unsupported.
- Poor hip stability on the saddle.
- Poor glute control.
- An over-reach to the bars and rounded shoulders as the centre of gravity is moved back.
- Compromised bike control due to poor weight bias and locked out arms.

What started as an uncomfortable saddle has now cascaded into a painful back and neck, as well as diminished power and efficiency.

And this mostly happens under the rider's conscious radar. Typically, when we film a rider and show them what we think is going on, it provokes a torrent of introspection about rides or events that ended with a poor performance, due to unmanageable discomfort. Once again, it's worth reiterating that the bike is an abstract environment, so none of us, not even bike fitters, have an innate capacity to deconstruct this for ourselves. We generally never discuss posture and pedalling technique until the athlete is in their theoretically best position for their discipline, such as track, TT, road, mountain biking, criterium or hill climbing. Only then will a positive change in posture result in a similarly constructive adaptation in function and power and comfort.

The first question we ask when a client tells us about back pain is to enquire if the pain is one-sided or symmetrical. This is important because if the pain is felt only on one side, it means the bike is acting upon the body in an unequal way.

The second and third questions are whether the pain goes away when they stop cycling, and is it only cycling that causes the pain? If they answer yes to both, we can assume for the moment that the interface with their bike is the probable underlying cause, and as such a review of their cycling biomechanics is entirely rational. If they answer no to either or both of those questions, we're much more circumspect. The bike may only be one part of a more fundamental issue and we strongly urge a referral to a physio or GP for further investigation. Other red flags are tingling or numbness down the backs of one or both legs, which may even extend into the foot. Generally speaking, it's a medical professional, not a bike fitter, who is needed at this point. The exception to this rule is when the client has a confirmed diagnosis of a problem, such as a herniated disc or sciatica, piriformis syndrome, etc; and our job is to work under medical direction to offload the affected structures as best we can so the individual can stay active and healthy. It is, however, our opinion that the bike is probably not the right environment for any neural issue that relates to the spine, because of the possibility that unguarded spinal flexion could make things worse.

If the back pain is symmetrical and quickly diminishes after cycling, the causes are easier to predict:

- The saddle is too high, introducing too much tension into the posterior-chain – which can be felt in the QL muscle. Fix: Lower the saddle and/or shorten the crank.
- The saddle is too far back or too far forward, making the rider unstable. Fix: Reset the relationship between the tip of the saddle and the bottom bracket.
- Incorrect saddle. This can leave the athlete inappropriately supported and therefore unstable, which can be felt in the QL as they try to stabilise the trunk. Fix: Find a more suitable saddle that suits the athlete's pelvis construction.
- The handlebars are too low for the athlete's physical conditioning, which can be felt in the lower lumbar and into the mid- and upper back. An aggressive cycling position has to be earned with exceptional core conditioning and flexibility. Professional cyclists earn that slammed stem with hours in the gym. Expect the vertical drop from your saddle to your bars to change with your weight, flexibility, and trunk/core conditioning.
- The athlete is pulling up on the pedals and overworking the hip flexors, which can be felt around the lower to mid-back where the hip flexors attach. Fix: Retrain the pedalling action to only push down (see p. 194).
- The crank is too long, creating an unsustainable acute angle between the spine and femur at the top of the pedal stroke, which can be felt in the lower lumbar through to the mid-back. Fix: Shorten the crank.

- Cycling posture is poor, with the pelvis rotated too far forwards (which is rare unless you're a yoga instructor) or too far back (far more likely). Fix: Strength and conditioning to support a sustainable neutral spine posture on your bike, which in turn will give your spine protection by encouraging your back and trunk muscles to switch on when you're cycling.
- Poor foot posture and control. Fix: Fix the foot first. Just as sciatica can be felt in the foot, so a misalignment of the foot can travel up to the back (although this is rare). Rare but not unknown.

If the back pain is asymmetrical but quickly diminishes after cycling, the causes and fixes can be a little harder to hunt down. The first thing we check is the bike itself:

- Are the cranks the same length? This is rare, but occasionally they aren't – bike companies and bike mechanics sometimes make mistakes.
- Is the saddle lower on one side due to a buckled rail or wear to the padding? This is surprisingly common.
- Are the cleats set up the same? Is one cleat more worn than the other? Inevitably, this is the case.
- Are the handlebars bent? And the levers level? Is the stem out of line? Again, these are common issues.

Assuming that the bike and all its components are correct and well aligned, the focus will move to the athlete and how they functionally interface with their bike.

- Functional or anatomical difference in leg length. (This is tested on the physio plinth and reflected in different knee-extension angles using motion-capture.) It will cause pain anywhere in the lower-mid or upper back, though this is most likely around the QL, which could overwork to stabilise the pelvis. Fix: Possible temporary stack, change the cleat position fore and aft.

- Relative tightness or shortness in one hamstring, calf or hip flexor can pull unevenly on the pelvis/spine while on the bike. Fix: Strength and conditioning to address the tightness, as well as a possible temporary stack and/or cleat position to partially compensate.

- Scoliosis can be a significant structural spinal asymmetry – it is just a question of degree. Fix: The bike position should be set up conservatively in terms of reach and drop so as not to stress the structures around the spine. It may also be necessary to set one shifter higher and further back on the shorter side.

- Pedalling dynamics. Sometimes the athlete is mostly symmetrical, but the asymmetry is introduced via their motor-patterning. For example, excessive dorsiflexion on one foot and plantar flexion on the other: through uneven movement at the ankle joint, one side is now significantly shorter than the other. The dysfunction in the pedal stroke is often an unhelpful legacy adaption from a previous injury that was perhaps not rehabbed properly. The functionally shorter side will probably be the side with lower lumbar pain, but the functionally longer side may experience hip pain due to the closed angle at the top of the pedal stroke. These can be frustratingly insoluble problems to fix, even when the asymmetry is pointed out to the client. We recently worked with a high-level, midlife fell runner who had switched to road riding, but was suffering from lower back pain due to mismatched pedalling motor-patterning. We fitted his bike with flat pedals and shorter cranks to try to alter his proprioception, while osteopath Alex Fugallo taped from his heel to his calf on the dorsiflexing side to try to make his exaggerated pedalling dynamics conscious. He also had a treating physio, who worked alongside in support. It took a few months and a lot of hard work, but he was able to relearn a more symmetrical pedalling style and resume high-level training again – without back pain.

Upper body pain – neck, shoulders, arms and hands

We've always thought of the cycling body in motion, viewed from the side, divided into thirds. The lower body is responsible for power production and transmission. The trunk's role is foundation and stabilisation. The upper body's part in this cycling drama is control and comfort. It's helpful to characterise yourself in this tri-segmented way, to the extent that cycling involves you being umbilically joined to an unyielding machine that will exert specific demands and stresses on your body as you produce power.

If the upper body is to provide fine machine control, while maintaining resilience to long kilometres in the saddle over a variety of terrain, the trunk/core area must deliver a vital 'dissociative role' from your lower body engine room. If your posture on the bike is ideal and your trunk/core muscles are engaged, you'll have a strong platform for your driving glutes, quads and calf extensor muscles, as well as a trunk that is positively braced in its active forward stance, allowing your upper body to relax in order to steer, brake and maintain control should you hit a pothole, or brush elbows or handlebars with another rider.

In our experience, most hand, arm, shoulder and neck problems relate to incorrect bike set-up or posture, which compromises an optimal lower body/trunk/upper body engagement/loading relationship.

Remember, none of this is ever fixed – just because you had a big drop from the saddle to the bars when you were 25 doesn't mean that you should when you're 55 – you could be heavier, less flexible, have a weaker core/trunk or even be carrying an injury that you didn't have 30 years ago. Here are the most common issues that we see:

1   Upper trapezius pain. This is most often described by clients as burning neck pain, which can be worse on one side or the other. Possible causes and fixes:

- Handlebars are too low and/or are too far away. Fix: Bring the bars up and back to encourage a more neutral shoulder angle (start with 90 degrees).

- Poor posture. The posterior rotation of the pelvis, also known as slouching, can cause the neck to hyperextend to maintain forward vision. Hyperextension will increase the loading on the trapezius muscles. Fixes: Cultivate a neutral spine to control neck posture. Also check your position on the bike – having the bars too far away and/or too low can encourage you to rotate your pelvis back to shift your centre of gravity away from the fall to the bar. Again, this will be an unconscious and unhelpful shift – when the there is too much weight on the hands and arms, one of the only things a rider can do is rotate the pelvis back to shift their body mass back. This will tend to switch off both core and glute activity, which is undesirable.

- Poor saddle contact. If the saddle contact is wrong, you may find that you're rotating your hips back and away from frontal saddle pressure. This happens often with female athletes. Fix: It may be necessary to level the saddle or adjust to up to -2 or -3 degrees nose-down (never nose-up), or even revise the saddle choice.

- If none of these fixes work, then it may not be the trapezius causing pain. Instead, it could be neural or neuromuscular. We would make an onward referral to a medical professional for evaluation and treatment.

2   Overloading through arms, causing tension and pain. This can be on one side but is more common on both, and arms may also lock out as a response. Possible causes and fixes:

- The drop from the saddle to the bars isn't sustainable for the level of trunk/core conditioning. Fix: Lift the handlebars until a 20-degree bend at the elbow can be comfortably maintained.

- Work on trunk/core strength and conditioning to increase your tolerance to the drop from the saddle to the bar. As a general rule of thumb we recommend starting by doing a plank tolerance test, using the following starting set-up guides. Remember, you have to earn your position! If you cannot ride comfortably on the drops when you're riding at pace, then the front end of the bike is probably too low:
  Plank test: 0 < 30 seconds: handlebars level or above saddle
  30 seconds – 1 minute: 0–4cm saddle-to-bar drop
  1 minute – 90 seconds: 4–6cm saddle-to-bar drop
  90 seconds – 2 minutes: 6–8cm saddle-to-bar drop
  > 2 minutes: 8–12cm saddle-to-bar drop

- The saddle is set too far forwards in relation to the bottom bracket, moving your centre of gravity too far forward and loading up through your arms. Fix: Recalibrate and reset your fore/aft saddle position.

- The handlebars are too far away, causing the arms to stretch too far. Fix (a pretty simple one, this): Shorten the stem or use a shorter reach handlebar.

- An inappropriately wide saddle is causing you to shuffle forwards, looking for a narrower part of the saddle. This will also move your centre of gravity forwards and possibly load the arms. Fix: Get a more suitable saddle.

- Poor technique. Some folk just get lazy and decide to lock out their arms rather than use their core/upper-body strength. Fix: Your homework is to try introducing that 20-degree bend at the elbow when you ride more of the time – channel the fall forward into the back/trunk and core structures.

3   Pain, numbness, or pins and needles in the hands. This can be felt in one or both hands but it's often felt particularly on one side. Some ultraendurance riders struggle with the numbness days or even weeks after a big event like Paris-Brest-Paris. Possible causes and fixes:

- Pain and/or tingling in the little and ring fingers, caused by a possible compression of the ulnar nerve, which innervates (supplies with nerves,) the fourth finger and half of the third finger. Fix: Offload the ulnar nerve by raising the bars, increasing core/trunk engagement, wearing more heavily padded gloves and/or changing the handlebar shape.

- Pain and/or tingling in the thumb and first three fingers – these are innervated by the median nerve. The same advice as above applies – the area needs to be offloaded or unweighted.

- Ulnar/median nerve compression. The ulnar and median nerves track down the arm from the upper spine. Sometimes an issue with the nerve root in the upper back can cause referred pain down the arm. The quality of the pain is generally different than simple compression at the hand (it's deeper and more neural) and there's often accompanying pain high up in the upper back/neck area. Fix: Referral to a physio/medical professional for diagnosis and treatment. If you were advised that you can ride through treatment, the bike position and posture must be amended to lessen the pressure at the wrist and hand. The neck and upper back posture must also be kept neutral to prevent the issue progressing further. It may well be that cycling and the probable incidence of spinal flexion isn't advised for a while.

4   Shoulder pain or problems. Like the knee and hip, the shoulder is a synovial joint and, like the hip, consists of a ball and socket. The shoulder is the most mobile joint in our body and one of the most painful if it goes wrong. It's sometimes hard for athletes

to discern whether the pain derives from the shoulder joint itself or from the trapezius that traverses out along the collar bone and shoulder blade (scapula). If the pain is thought to be directed towards the shoulder joint itself, there are a few adjustments to try. Possible underlying causes and potential fixes on the bike could be:

- Make sure that the hand and wrist is right underneath the centre of the acromioclavicular (AC) joint. Many riders use bars that are too wide because they unwittingly measure their shoulder width from outside to outside. If the bar is too wide, the rider may find they are rotating their wrists inwards to effectively narrow the handlebar to make it more comfortable. Fix: Measure from the centre of the shoulder joint and use an appropriate-width bar.

- Using a handlebar that's too narrow will possibly introduce tension around the whole shoulder complex. Using a handlebar that's too narrow can be worse than using a handlebar that's too wide. Fix: As above, measure from the centre of the shoulder joint and use an appropriate-width bar.

The perfect pedal stroke

Along with chapter 3, this section may be the most important one in the whole book. Firstly, because pedalling poorly is inefficient and can also cause pain and injury. And secondly, because the whole subject of the ideal pedal stroke is surrounded in unhelpful mythology that refuses to die. So to get going, let's touch on the Myth of the Upstroke. The upstroke is cycling's Flat Earth movement, the only difference being that the upstroke's continuing proliferation makes it more mainstream. The Upstrokers are still out there, unwittingly pedalling their poor advice. The notion of a circular pedal stroke is still being propagated in respected books and articles, as well as by influential companies who seek to help you achieve such a thing by using one of their products. The concept of the upstroke seems credible for a few seductive but bogus reasons:

- By pedalling in circles, you use all your muscles through the whole cycle.
- By pulling up you can pedal through the dead spot at the top and bottom of the pedal stroke.
- You clip in precisely to facilitate pulling up as well as pushing down on the pedal.
- It feels faster when you do it, doesn't it?
- Pedalling up makes you smoother – you turn from a V-twin into a turbine electric motor.
- Being smooth must be more efficient than being lumpy, right?

These are attractive and reasonable theories but they are also totally false. Moreover, they impede countless riders' efficiency, health and quiet enjoyment of the simple act of pedalling their bicycles.

Let's deconstruct this most ubiquitous and damaging of assumptions. The concept of the upstroke appeals to our common sense – we use lots of muscles to move our legs, and it stands to reason that we can pedal faster if we use more of them, more of the time. What's not to like about that biomechanical scenario? Except, as I keep pointing out, we're perfectly evolved to walk and run, not pedal a bicycle. When we run, we produce power to move forwards only when we have actual ground contact. Great runners have ground contact for only around 200 milliseconds per stride. In fact, reducing ground contact time (GCT) is considered to be an advanced technique for increasing cadence, efficiency and speed. During GCT we use hip extension, knee extension and ankle plantar flexors to propel ourselves forwards and free of the ground into the float phase (when we are suspended in mid-air). Our powerful extensor muscles – glutes, quads and calves – have evolved perfectly to provide this explosive extension in a fraction of a second as we toe off the ground. During the float phase the hip and knee flex and the foot dorsiflexes (pulls the toes up) as the leg is lifted and drawn forwards, ready for ground contact. All of this flexion and dorsiflexion occurs with air contact only – there's no ground contact. The hip and knee extensors act upon the weight of the limb against gravity only. As a consequence, the hip flexors are a relatively tiny muscle group compared to the hip extensors (glutes). The former is, in a sense, a postural muscle and the latter is your dominant bipedal propulsive muscle, which explodes us free of the ground. When you see the hip flexor and hip extensor side by side, it's clear which muscle we need to engage and which one we need to be mindful that we don't overuse. The hip flexor functions in a restricted and compacted space and can easily become irritated and inflamed because of a dysfunctional pedal stroke. We've worked with many athletes over the years, including professional cyclists, who have experienced chronic problems related to hip flexor overdominance on one or both sides (normally one side). Pulling up when you're pedalling is the running equivalent of attempting to increase GCT by recruiting a tiny postural muscle and repurposing it as a power generator. It's both futile and potentially harmful. By the way, runners often try to reduce GCT to make themselves faster!

Now, in case you have any lingering doubts on the subject of the upstroke, the research says, don't pull up. Our friend and colleague Dr Jeffrey Broker (Associate Professor, University of Colorado at Colorado Springs) proved with his groundbreaking research what many of has had long suspected – the upstroke is a distracting non-event.

Broker's research was predicated on a piece of technology that was specially designed and built for the research – the force pedal, which could measure forces being applied to it in all directions, including an upwards force on the backside of the pedal stroke. Broker's research evaluated a hundred elite and professional cyclists by geographically mapping their in-time force application onto the pedals as they rode in a controlled environment. Dr Broker's research proved that pedalling 'was a completely non-circular event – the motion is circular, but the force application is far from circular'.

The output of the research was pretty binary and what we had suspected – power in the stroke was derived from extensor (glute, quad and calf) activity in the power phase (downstroke) and nothing was being produced during the recovery phase (upstroke). Dr Broker's data clearly shows that all the way through the upstroke there is, in fact, negative pressure on the pedal, where the uphill leg is pushing back the wrong way on the pedal due to the effects of gravity. Dr Broker talks about those athletes who consciously thought they were positively contributing to the upstroke: 'There's the sensation of lifting and pulling, but you don't do it fast enough to get out of the way of the pedal.' The conclusion is clear – the world's best athletes, even when they tried, couldn't positively contribute to a meaningful power delivery during the recovery phase.

The study included a powerful rider who was criticised for his 'mashing' pedal technique, at a time when all coaches in Europe and the US venerated a smooth, circular pedalling technique (they even had a name for it, souplesse). The rider was a young Lance Armstrong, who smacked the pedals in anger rather than caressed them delicately like Stephen Roche. At the same time, Greg LeMond, three-time Tour de France winner and technical innovator, was exhorting us to pull back at the bottom of the pedal arc, as if we were scraping dog poo off our shoes. It was always a lively topic during training sessions – we all wanted to be Roche rather than Armstrong but we also paid attention to LeMond, because he was first to everything. But even in our little team I remember that it was the mashers who seemed to win most of the races. Jay, by popular consent, was the complete pedaller, but it was Mark, clubbing the pedals into submission, who would most often be last man standing on race day.

There was a fad at the time, and possibly still is in some circles (excuse the pun), that single-leg pedal drills would improve your pedalling mechanics. We couldn't disagree more – single-leg pedal drills will likely embed poor motor-patterning by forcing you to overuse weak, postural, flexor muscles during the recovery phase. Even worse are the independently moving cranks, where you're forced to control every movement of each crank minutely and individually – but to what dividend or benefit? Where is the evidence? It can also destabilise the pelvic/saddle contact.

Equally we don't really understand some pedalling software attached to some training technology, such as Wattbike. Which muscle groups are Wattbike trying to activate with its Peanut and Sausage techniques, and for what specific aim? We're truly interested – it's always fascinating to learn new approaches and philosophies.

It's thought by some biomechanists and cycling physios (and us, in fact) that we simply don't have the available neural RAM or proprioceptive ability to be able to generate any meaningful force on the upstroke at anything approaching full cadence and full power. We simply didn't evolve to pedal with a flexed hip and spine and still try to yank up on the ground – it's an unnatural act. Try it for yourself while seated to evaluate how it feels. You don't have to be on your bike; just push down on one knee with both hands. Now try lifting that knee with all your force against the downward force of your hands. Alternatively, while on the bike on a gentle incline, try pedalling by only pulling up for one minute (not to be tried by anyone with an ongoing hip issue). This should be enough to convince you that the hip flexors evolved to be used against fresh air and not a pedal.

It should be clear that we possess neither the hardware nor software to positively contribute to total pedal forces via an upstroke. Our work with professional cyclists has also taught us a couple of other points about the application of pedal force. Firstly, that professional cyclists seem to have relatively short and dynamic pedal strokes, meaning they produce huge amounts of power over a very small range, centred around the crank at 90 degrees – or parallel to the ground. They also reduce the effective length (circumference) of the pedal stroke as they increase power output. Contemporary professional cyclists, set up in a progressive, modern position, are far from pedalling in fluid circles – they are staccato, ballistic, watt factories.

Secondly, professional cyclists seem to deviate from their functional and dynamic/extension style, and start pulling up on the pedals, only when they are injured or are recovering from injury. The pulling up is almost always an unconscious and unhelpful adaption. We also see this with amateur cyclists. Pulling up is a destabilising pedalling dysfunction.

Pedalling paracetamol

A technique that we frequently use, with both professional and amateur clients, if we suspect they are pulling up or 'compensating', is to ask them to pedal on a flat pedal wearing a running shoe rather than cycling shoe. And tracking the pedal scan, as well as their subjective emotional response, is fascinating. Most often we see the pedal scan settle back down to dynamic equilibrium as soon as they are unclipped. Similarly, we see their faces relax as their hip and back pain unwinds and dissipates – we call this 'pedalling paracetamol'. Sometimes the simplest and cheapest fixes are the best. Please feel free to use this technique yourself if you've any kind of cycling pain – it's both a diagnostic tool and a retraining tool. It's immensely powerful, and free.

The ankling myth

Another hangover from the 'back in the day' era – if we weren't being harangued about pulling back and up, we were being told to 'drop our ankles' when pedalling. Most of us never stopped and questioned why transferring power through a moving joint could ever be a desirable thing. What other sport or power posture involves dropping the heel (aside from showjumping on a horse)? It was virtually unopposed that ankling or dorsiflexing the foot was a desirable attribute, maybe because so many of our heroes exhibited this behaviour. But let's turn it on its head: I contend that the reason why many of our heroes ankled when they pedalled was actually rooted in mainly negative underlying causes – saddles were too low, they had tight hip-in-flexion ranges, they were climbing in gears that were too high or they were using cranks that were too long. Put all of those together and they had little choice but to excessively drop the heel at the top of the pedal stroke to create requisite space for the crank to clear the hip. Now it's no longer necessary to flex the ankle to the same degree because both professional and amateur athletes are better conditioned in terms of flexibility, and routinely use shorter cranks and better gearing, and sit on a saddle that is less set back behind the bottom bracket (in other words, has a forward centre of gravity). This results in a more efficient and comfortable transfer of power.

The cadence myth

Lance Armstrong produced huge amounts of power for many reasons – some of them legal. But cadence was effect and not cause. We know that he started as a lumpy masher and not a turbine spin dryer. Armstrong, as in so many things, did start a new debate about cadence, where 100rpm became the new standard we should aim for. In our experience, lots of people can hold 100rpm with a properly functioning, comfortable and sustainable pedal stroke, and just as many cannot. You shouldn't berate yourself or try to hold 100rpm if it feels strange or uncomfortable. If you try to maintain an unnaturally high cadence, there are likely compensatory consequences such as instability on the saddle and dysfunction in the pedalling action as you reflexively try (and fail) to get your foot out the way of the uphill pedal. Better to consciously sit back on the pedal stroke a little and ensure that the power is concentrated around extension in the downstroke. We don't like quoting arbitrary limits, but 80rpm is perhaps a usable minimum for riding on a flat road with no headwind. That may be the point that either your technique, bike position, crank length or flexibility/conditioning have become operational impediments – for example, the saddle is too low, the crank too long, or you are tight around hips. You would probably be advised to review all the above before trying to propel your cadence more positively into rocket-fuelled Armstrong territory.

So, let's review the perfect pedal stroke and how you get it. The message is clear – simplest is always best. As an aside, we often see absolute beginners on flat pedals and world champions who are clipped in with similar pedal scan shapes (but totally different power outputs). That's to say, poor pedalling technique is generally either consciously learned or an unconscious adaption. Pedalling doesn't need to be thought about. You'll do it correctly if the context is right and you don't get in its way. In review, here are the fundamentals:

- Almost all the power is concentrated in the downstroke. The upstroke isn't something that needs to be consciously worked on or thought about, and to do so is a waste of time.
- The heel should stay positively angled all through the pedal stroke. If this isn't the case, check saddle height, crank length, cadence, calf strength and technique.
- Not everyone can, or should, pedal at 100rpm or more. Find the cadence that works for you. If you want to increase your cadence, improve your core/trunk conditioning, increase flexibility, shorten your cranks and review your bike position.
- Use some pedalling paracetamol. If in doubt, unclip as both a diagnostic and retraining tool. It could change your life (well, at least your pedalling).

Whenever your bike has ceased to be your best friend and has, of late, started to hurt you, it's worth remembering a few of our totemic bike guiding principles. The most important being that *humans did not evolve to ride bicycles!* Despite how much we love them, bikes are a Victorian daydream preserved in aspic for well over a century because of a speciation event involving the UCI, path dependence and a huge dose of nostalgia. We love their shape, links with our own childhoods and, of course, powerful romantic associations to cycle sport. But it is worth pointing out that when Mark Cavendish wanted to unleash the world's most formidable explosive power, he did so by deliberately pulling his body forwards out of the constraints the Victorian biomechanists conceived for him, until his whole torso was over the front of the bike as he snapped back on the downstroke. His speed came despite the architecture of the bicycle, and not because of it. That was part of his genius. He had worked out that you can't release 1800 watts or more sitting down on a saddle like you're sitting at a desk. Cavendish wasn't the first sprinter to adopt this posture, but in our opinion he was its finest exponent. He also had the huge advantage that as he pulled himself into his aggressive sprinting posture, he was also lowering his frontal silhouette to the wind and therefore made himself more aerodynamically efficient. Bicycles are beautiful objects and are especially beguiling to us staccato bipeds, for their ability to transform potential into kinetic energy. I was a physically discombobulated kind of a kid – I hated football and running and failed to catch every ball ever thrown at me. I couldn't wait for school to end so I could jump on my bike and feel the energy flow again. I mostly still feel like that today. But that 'flow' requires more conscious thought, preparation and conditioning every year, if it's to be maintained. The bicycle ultimately is a dictator of control points and a physical limiter of movement. You feel free but you're not free. Despite my harsh criticisms, I adore bicycles and I find it impossible ever to get rid of any of them – all our adventures are written in the patina on the saddle scuffs and paint chips. But as a bike fitter I also know the design was fortunate to make it out of the 19th century mostly unchallenged, never mind the 20th.

So, go back to first principles when your bike doesn't feel right. Start by releasing yourself from the machine by pedalling standing up or taking a dose of pedalling paracetamol and not clipping in. Release the kinetic chains and move outside the bike's constraints. And then start reviewing the relationship of your changing and possibly asymmetrical biomechanics with your bicycle's immutable and probably very symmetrical form. Remember: if it becomes a tug of war, the Victorian contraption will always win.

6

BIKE, WHAT BIKE?

In my experience, buying a new car is generally a profoundly disappointing experience, whereas getting a new bike is a promise of adventure and a further opportunity to enrich your body and soul. Riding your bike is intrinsically a great thing for your physical and mental health. The same cannot be said for driving a car. Where there is a similarity, however, is in the head/heart dichotomy. Your head politely suggests a Volvo estate while your heart shrieks Maserati. The same is true for a new bike, but the implications can be more profound, as you push your body to achieve more, in an environment (i.e. bike position) that doesn't necessarily support your endeavours. Both the head and the heart are important lodestars when buying something as emotive as a bicycle – hopefully this brief guide can help you recognise which of your two vital organs should be leading the debate.

If I were writing this 40 years ago, there wouldn't have been many decisions to make, other than colour. Your bike would almost certainly have been fabricated from traditional lugged steel, using hand-built wheels, friction gears and toe clips. Working out the correct geometry and fit would have involved the timeworn process of copious teeth sucking and chin stroking. Most post-war competition bikes in Britain were made from Reynolds venerable and magnificent 531c tubing. Reynolds 531 tubing was the product of a continent between two world wars, and the emergence of an increasingly sophisticated aircraft industry that was perceived as a way of winning wars – or, at least, not losing them. 531 was sophisticated seamless steel tubing that was made stronger, lighter and stiffer by alloying it with a combination of manganese and molybdenum. It was a truly remarkable and magical material in the 1930s, and went on to win multiple Tour de France victories (24 at the last count). Incidentally, the Dutch rider Joop Zoetemelk won the 1980 Tour de France for team Ti-Raleigh using a heat-treated version of 531, called Reynolds 753. I have ridden thousands of miles on Reynolds 531c-framed bikes over the decades and the ride is astoundingly springy and satisfying. Competition bikes 40 years ago (these were the days of the Austin Metro and Vauxhall Cavalier, remember) fell into a few very discreet silos. There were road bikes, cyclo-cross bikes and very bespoke one-off lo-pro time trial bikes, and that was about it. There were no mountain bikes, aero or gravel bikes. These categories had not yet been invented.

So much has changed in the last 40 years – the industry barely pauses to draw breath before it either rearranges the deck chairs or simply flings them over the side. There's now a kaleidoscope of design and technology available to the cycling enthusiast. What follows is an incomplete and shamelessly biased assessment of what you may need, and what you may not.

Fit first: Join the dots

The first thing you should do if you're contemplating your first bike, or an addition to your existing collection, is to book a bike fit with a professional who has been recommended to you, preferably by more than one person. A bike that's too big or too small, or conceptually wrong, will never feel functional or comfortable. You'll always struggle to progress and reach your goals on a bike that neither fits nor suits its intended purpose. A bike fit should be your time under the spotlight – it should be fun, informative and relevant. You should be asked a little about your history (riding, sporting, injury) but also about your aspirations – what are you going to do with your new bike? The bike fitter's job is to join the dots between how you present yourself on the day as an athlete, and your stated goals, whether that's to ride around a park or around the world. This may well be your first time being professionally assessed – it will not be theirs. It is important to understand that bike fitting is a process, and not an event. Your focus, fitness and goals will change with time's arrow. I had a client who arrived at 64kg and appeared 10 years later at 128kg. I knew what a formidable athlete he had been on a bike before work and family preoccupied him, and I therefore trusted the weight loss and fitness programme he had self-prescribed. I knew that I would be well-advised to put the bike and bike position slightly ahead of how he appeared on any one day. Last I heard he was back hitting the high numbers, if not riding around the globe as he once had.

There's never a shortage of opinions or advice in the world of cycling. Folk with good intentions (often due to cognitive bias) lead you down a road that may be right for them but not necessarily for you. The best advice I always think is the kind you pay for – because it comes with both experience and a duty of care. Our own cognitive bias is that you should seek out a bike fitter for every new bike.

Spoilt for choice

Recent technology shifts have satisfyingly blurred the edges of the road, gravel, cyclo-cross and aero categories into a theoretical Venn diagram that's stuffed with rich and overlapping possibilities.

Disc brakes are here to stay, whether you like them or not. It's worth saying that conventional rim brakes reached their peak innovation around 2014. Post 2014 most manufacturers of bikes and components have chosen to redirect their R&D dollars towards frames, components, wheels, forks and tyres that are all compatible with disc brakes. Braking on the rims was never a good idea and cars stopped doing it in the 1920s – we had to wait for almost a hundred years for road bikes to follow suit. The only downside to disc brakes on a bike is that they currently add about 400g to the overall weight. In addition to the enhanced stopping power and control, the other huge benefit of discs is how they have liberated the architecture of the bicycle frame. Caliper brakes limited tyre size, and tyre size in turn limited your use horizon. Free yourself of calipers, and the real estate gained can be usefully filled with adventure potential. No longer do you need to choose between road and off-road, or gravel and aero – you can get it all in one bike that does everything. Your first task when you're contemplating a bike is to ensure that you put your money where the miles are – start by sitting down and sketching out your perfect riding landscape and then edge your bike in that direction. For example, if you want to ride:

1   Mostly long road miles
2   Occasional tracks and trails
3   Frequently in the winter
4   Occasional organised events and rides
5   Trips and events in the mountains in the summer
6   Very infrequent races at pace,

go for a bike with:

1   Geometry that favours long hours riding on the road
2   Comfortable ride quality on longer rides
3   Clearance for 35mm trail tyres
4   Mudguard braze-ons, to make winter riding pleasant
5   Light enough weight for events and riding in the mountains
6   Few aero credentials (but the bike should be fast enough for bunch rides).

There are dozens of road/gravel bikes that hit this brief. However, if you swapped the criteria around and put the aero requirement nearer or at the top of your list, the choice becomes more difficult and the trade-offs more stark. That's to say, the rounder the tube, the stiffer and stronger it is. Bike manufacturers are compelled to add additional carbon fibre as they draw the tubes into the larger-profile aerofoil shapes, in order to maintain the same overall stiffness in the ride. The effect of oversizing the tubes and increasing the carbon material makes the frame both heavier and less comfortable. Which may be acceptable if you're a rider with a basement full of watts that you want to spend and can therefore pay your way into a full aero dividend. But it's less compelling if you don't produce as much power and can't easily access the speeds where aero becomes marginally more important, that is to say generally above 32km/h. Now you're just riding a heavier, less comfortable bike, at a slower pace, up a hill, just because it has an aero profile.

A 75kg rider who produces 400 watts may still be receiving an aero benefit even when the road has reached an 8 per cent gradient. In contrast, a 60kg rider who can access only 250 watts could lose any aerodynamic benefit once the road tilts up beyond 4 per cent. The smaller, less powerful rider may be better served with a broader shopping basket of criteria, where weight and ride quality occupy more prominence.

Going back to the brief – the aero criteria will be difficult to achieve if the other conditions of light weight, comfort and mudguard fittings are to be maintained. Finding your own personal bullseye requires a forensic level of preferencing, which is often best worked through with a professional, who is happy to flag up the difficult choices.

Sometimes a client comes in with a fixation on a certain model, and even size of bike. And during the Cyclefit process it becomes clear that this isn't likely to be a beneficial partnership, either because the bike doesn't fit their morphology or because the ride characteristics will not flatter their own skill levels and riding style. Questions that we ask are:

1   How confident are you cornering?
2   How confident are you descending at pace?
3   What aspects of your riding style would you like to improve?
4   Can you easily take one or both hands off the handlebars?

This is where you need to be honest with yourself. Maybe you lack confidence cornering, braking or descending and no matter how hard you work at it you don't seem to get any better. You certainly would benefit from instruction from a patient teacher, but you also need a bike that's going to give you confidence as you acquire new skills. We would recommend a bike with a particular geometry:

1   A lower bottom bracket to lower your overall centre of gravity and sit you deeper into the bike.
2   A longer chainstay and increased wheelbase to impart stability and a sense that the bike will steer itself down a hill.
3   A slacker head angle to slow the steering down a little.
4   A longer head tube, so you don't feel like you're falling forwards onto your hands, a feeling that's exacerbated when descending at speed.

Sometimes geometry like the one described above is called 'endurance' or 'sportive' by bicycle companies – these new design platforms were influenced by the emergence of the bike fitting community over the last 10 to 15 years. Progressive bike companies invited us and our colleagues into project development meetings for new models. Until that point it was assumed that riders of all ages would ride in the same position as professional riders only half their age. Endurance geometry has been adopted by most bike companies now, because helps many riders function more effectively and safely on their bikes.

I remember riding a huge day in the Alps some years ago with Jules and a group of our clients. It was a matter of pride, in this company, to be perfectly calibrated to your machine. All our bikes were full-custom and designed in-house by Cyclefit – and the companies PARLEE, Seven, Serotta and Passoni were all represented. On the descent I tucked in behind our client, Tom, gathering speed as we fell towards the valley floor, thousands of feet below. Tom was an obsessional perfectionist in his outlook towards his training, equipment and, sensibly, his set-up on his bike. But as the others in the group disappeared down the mountain, it was clear something was wrong with Tom. We rode slower and slower as he hung onto the brakes – to the point where I rode past and flagged him to a stop. It transpired that a recent crash and injury had eroded his confidence, especially when descending. The custom geometry, which we had conceived together and designed, featured a steep head angle, ultra-short chainstays and a short headtube – it was a pure race bike. The problem was that while it perfectly fitted his morphology – all the knee, hip and shoulder angles were technically correct – it simply no longer reflected his current technical riding ability or helped to repair his shattered confidence. It was just the wrong bike for him on this mountain on this day. He continued to fight his bike through the entire trip as soon as the road pointed dramatically downwards, tiptoeing through the corners and comfort braking down the straights. Had we been designing a bike for a client recovering from a crash and injury, the bike would have looked and ridden very differently. In this moment Tom needed a bike with a stable, low centre of gravity, detailed above, to help him rebuild his confidence and technique. It is what we arranged as soon as we returned to London.

Sometimes we have clients who want a bike that's technically wrong for them, but they want it anyway. 'I'm 50 years old, the fittest I have ever been – so if not now, when?' We hear this frequently. Ten years ago, we would have been more purist and possibly even tried to talk them out of it. Now we see their point, and it's a very fair one – we'll try to help realise their dream, but under certain provisos:

1   The bike must carefully calibrated – crank length, bar width, stem length, seat post layback, must all be carefully considered.
2   It shouldn't be the only bike they ride. They should also have a bike that does fulfil their personal frame of reference – i.e. is technically correct with respect to the individual's flexibility and physical conditioning.

3   They should have a strategy to grow into the bike and 'earn their position'. This could be working on flexibility and strength to make them more resilient to the stresses of an aggressive position.

Click and regret

There cannot be many worse ideas than buying a bike on the internet (unless you know specifically, beyond any doubt, what you need). If you have recent bike fitting dimensions that have been translated for you into frame geometry and/or stack and reach, then of course you'll be better prepared. Otherwise you could be operating mostly on guesswork. We've seen so many nightmares in the last 10 years – riders bringing in bikes that they aren't enjoying riding because they just don't feel right or are causing pain. Sometimes the frame is the wrong size, sometimes the model they have bought doesn't suit them well, or the set-up is wrong. Often, it's all the above. Most online bike companies are indifferent to these problems, in the sense that they aren't offering the expertise to deal with the issues that arise when the relationship between a rider and their bike breaks down.

The bicycle is inherently a dictatorial environment – you don't get to make many choices about how you function when you're on it. The position of your hands, pelvis and movement of your feet on the pedals are all prescribed. The bike, by definition, will not adapt or yield at all – you alone will be doing all the adjusting to the new bike and position. The interface between you and your new bike is complex and worthy of ongoing consideration, which is often difficult when a bike arrives at your door in a big cardboard box.

It's immaterial

We live in a carbon universe. Most folk are either riding a carbon fibre bike or they want to be at some point in the future. It's a pretty compelling proposition – carbon is responsible for some of the lightest and stiffest frames available. And while we continue to worship the twin gods of stiff and light, carbon will continue its primacy. However, carbon isn't the only material in town, and it may be worth looking at the alternatives before you assume that your next bike just has to constructed from the holy fibres. We'll come back to the frankly miraculous qualities of modern carbon fibre but before we do, it's worth discussing the relative merits and drawbacks of bicycles that are made of metal.

There are three metals that bike frames are commonly made of – steel, aluminium and titanium. A certain amount of mystery, and therefore assumption, unfairly surrounds all of them. First off, they can all be excellent materials to make bicycles from, provided they fit into your intention and lifestyle. There are a few criteria that we should benchmark against to provide an objective analysis:

1   Density – or 'weight'
2   Young's modulus of elasticity – or 'stiffness'
3   Elongation – or 'stretchiness'
4   Fatigue strength – or resistance to cyclical load
5   Resilience – or toughness, to withstand the ravages of time, use and weather

There are other characteristics that we could throw in, but as a general basket of qualities that's not a bad start.

So now assume that we build three identical frames – all the tubes are identical in every way except one frame is made from steel, one from aluminium and one is made from titanium. And when I say identical, I mean even the tube wall diameters, shapes and profiles are exactly the same. How will the apparently identical frames differ from each other?

1   Density – the aluminium frame will be approximately one-third of the weight of the steel one. The titanium frame will be just over half the weight of the steel frame. On that one criterion

alone, aluminium comes first and titanium and steel languish behind in second and third place respectively.

2   Young's modulus of elasticity – the steel frame will be twice as stiff as the titanium frame and three times stiffer than the aluminium frame.

3   Elongation – this criterion is more important than it may seem because it measures what happens when you push and pull the material to breaking point. Here titanium goes into first place, steel into second and aluminium, which really takes great exception to being pushed around, firmly into third place.

4   Fatigue strength – this measures how the frame responds to repeated cyclical loading, like pedalling and braking and going over bumps. And the podium results from 'elongation' are repeated – titanium has the best cyclical load resistance; steel has the second; and aluminium a distant third again.

5   Resilience – which of the frames will be most resilient to the rigours of the real world? Steel frames will rust if the conditions are right, and to a certain extent aluminium frames will corrode. Both these can be somewhat mitigated with paint and, in steel's case, treatment within the frame itself. Titanium doesn't need paint and will not rust or degrade at all – it's completely inert. On paper at least, this is another victory for titanium.

What does our experiment tell us? That aluminium is the lightest, steel is the stiffest and titanium is the most resilient? In truth, this example is a dramatic oversimplification – we've eliminated any notion of creating designs specific to a material. Aluminium, for example, comes a poor third in every criteria other than density (or weight). However, aluminium is actually so far ahead of the other two metals in terms of lightness, that many of its other downsides can, and are, successfully sidestepped by good design and fabrication. For example, if you double the diameter of a tube you'll increase its stiffness eightfold. The fact that aluminium is so lacking in density implies that it's entirely possible to add extra material to specific tubing profiles, then dramatically oversize them, to create a frame that's still lighter and stiffer than steel and possibly even titanium. In addition, aluminium is relatively inexpensive as a design and construction resource – so not many frame-building materials can equal it in terms of bang for your buck. But you do have to like the ride – all that plumping up of the tube diameters does yield a very direct connection with the earth's crust. Not a problem if this is being mediated through a 38mm gravel tyre, but possibly distracting when experienced through a 25mm road tyre. I raced for two seasons on Cannondale CAAD3 and CAAD4 oversized aluminium race bikes in the mid-1990s and they were sensational for explosive short-circuit criteriums, where acceleration and power transfer were very important. But I would always prefer to switch to a steel or titanium bike for longer road races or training rides, both of which I found significantly less stiff and fatiguing.

Steel scores well in every category other than weight (and its propensity to rust if untreated). It's still, in many ways, the benchmark of stiffness, strength and resilience. And, lest we forget, steel has that iconic ride – it may be the stiffest natural material by volume but that's not how it rides at all, assuming the frame has been lovingly made. Steel is famous for having an addictive capture-and-release, power delivery. Press down, and it gives back with a sprung action. While this is no longer on trend in a carbon world, it's still very satisfying as an alternate flavour. Owning (or at least riding) a steel frame is almost a cycling a rite of passage – put yourself on the bikes of Simpson, Merckx and Fignon. To this day, I have ridden and raced many more miles on steel bikes than I have on any other material. I find it impossible to separate the charismatic and beguiling ride from all the attendant heritage and romance that surrounds this mythic metal. By the way, we had a client who rode almost 1.6 million kilometres on his steel bike – he measured it with an old-fashioned milometer attached to the front wheel. Frequently we would be racing in Scotland or Wales on a mountain bike course in the middle of nowhere and then we would see Chris cheering us on. He had ridden hundreds of miles to support the event and would then ride back home again.

From the mythic metal to the magical metal: titanium has been surrounded with an aura ever since frame builders began experimenting with raw material left over from the aerospace industry in the 1970s and '80s. Everyone knew the potential of this quixotic drab-coloured metal, but nobody could capture its essence in seven bicycle tubes. Most frames either failed, or just failed to inspire. Titanium's reputation as the most recalcitrant metal became entrenched in the bike industry's consciousness at a time when carbon's star was already rising. Steel was given 100 years to ferment to maturation, titanium was all over in a decade or two – the enfant terrible. But titanium is neither steel or aluminium. It won't easily submit or yield to form. It fights back, blunts tools and will just not tolerate welding unless conditions are surgical. Steel, and to a degree aluminium, are forgiving and inexpensive materials to work with, but titanium occupies the opposing end of the spectrum. This 'grey gold' rightly became the domain of specialists who made it their life's work to articulate its magical properties within the humble bicycle frame. In the right hands, titanium delivers a remarkable magic carpet ride that seems to defy the laws of physics. Moreover, because of its unparalleled fatigue strength, it has no defined lifespan. It also won't rust, degrade or even change its ride properties over decades and tens of thousands of miles. It's the Dorian Gray of bicycle materials.

So where does carbon fibre fit into the material landscape? There's no easy answer to that question because carbon fibre is a composite of load-bearing fibre strands organised by an epoxy matrix or glue. Moreover, carbon is now so highly evolved that there are multiple recipes to choose from – high-modulus carbon, which is the lightest and stiffest material, through to low modulus, which is many times heavier and more malleable. Most bikes use a combination of different grades and lay-ups, depending on the stress in a particular area. Carbon fibre is a bike designer's dream because they are no longer constrained by the shape and properties of metal and how it will fold into tubing. Furthermore, it's also advantageous to bike companies because producing quality bicycles quickly became a highly industrial process, as opposed to something that was constrained by the speed of craftspeople.

But back to the original question – how does carbon compare with steel, aluminium and titanium? Let's assume a highly developed frame from one of the major factories, using the optimal contribution of high-modulus material. Carbon would be even lighter than aluminium and probably even stiffer than our class leader, steel. If we introduce a new criteria – tensile strength, or literally how much force needs to be applied to rip a material apart, measured in kilograms per square inch (kis) – then carbon would potentially outperform steel, titanium and aluminium. So carbon scores three first places for lightness, stiffness and strength – surely this is game over? Carbon is technically a remarkable material – nothing comes close in respect of stiffness to weight and weight. But it doesn't have great ductility numbers (the ability to be drawn without breaking), meaning it doesn't like to be stretched. Neither is it particularly resilient or resistant to being knocked and bumped – if, for example a stone bounces up from the road and hits the underside of the downtube sufficiently hard to breach the gelcoat or the weave structure underneath.

To sum up, all materials have their individual characteristics, which in turn are applicable to how we like to ride. We could all probably easily justify one of each depending on the weather, event or even our mood. Here is a quick assessment of each material's relative strengths and weaknesses:

- Steel – has a classic intuitive ride, it's resilient, beautiful and can last a million miles. But it's comparatively heavy and can rust.
- Aluminium – is very light and has superb bang for your buck but oversized tubing can make the ride quality a little harsh. Also, it can corrode and has potential longevity issues.

- Titanium – has a unique ride quality and potentially limitless lifespan. It's also stronger and tougher than every other material here, and is best for frequent travellers and fliers. However, it's difficult to work with, so the best titanium frames are very expensive, and always will be.
- Carbon – has unrivalled lightness, stiffness and tensile strength scores and it can be designed into any shape you like, unlike metal. It's also easy to mass-produce. However, it's not that durable and has a binary ride experience in the sense that it is the quickest to respond to any input – acceleration, braking, steering.

Once you've selected your ideal frame material, based on your planned riding, you just have to select the right genre of bike. The following is an outline of the different choices you have:

- Road bike – the classic all-rounder, which will handle any kind of road on any kind of day. Typically used for training or racing. Neutral geometry and handling. Now almost certain to have clearances for 28mm or even 32mm tyres. Winter road bikes may have lower bottom bracket heights and longer chainstays to facilitate mudguards and 32mm tyres.
- Aero road bike – a comparatively new genre, aero road bikes are for people who have forsaken all criteria other than outright speed. An aero road bike has deeper aerofoils on the main tubes and tighter clearances. They can theoretically save you 15–40 watts of power, but only at speeds above 30km/h. The faster you ride, the bigger the dividend you get. Their primary problem is that they are often heavier and less composed on poor roads and in big winds.
- Cyclo-cross bike – the classic crosser was designed for up to an hour's riding in virtual mud criteriums. It featured high bottom brackets for log clearance, a maximum of one bottle cage, an

open frame design (no sloping top tubes) to allow easy portage (carrying), and cable routing to allow riders to shoulder their bikes. The cross frame has been made somewhat redundant by the emergence of the gravel bike, but it's still one of the most fun ways to spend an autumn morning riding among the leaves.

- Gravel bike – who knew we needed another category? Gravel bikes are the natural intersection of cross and road. They have bigger clearances than cross bikes and usually have a lower bottom bracket for off-road stability. They often have at least two or even three bottle cage mounts to allow expedition riding and often the option to switch from a 700c wheel with a 40mm tyre to a 650b wheel with a mountain bike knobbly tyre. Gravel bikes have swallowed up the market with their all-round greatness and versatility. There's very little they can't do well – except perhaps ride on the track. Jules raced his Open U.P. in three different disciplines in one week – a cyclo-cross race, a road race and a mountain bike race.

- Track bike – the purest, stripped back version of a modern bicycle; no brakes, a single fixed gear (meaning that if you're moving, then you're pedalling), no bottle cages. They are light, furiously quick and made to ride around in circles at your theoretical maximum. Try a track bike at least once in your life.

- Aero or TT (time trial) bike – drag=V^2, which means that aerodynamic drag increases as a square of your speed. The faster you ride, the more important aerodynamics are. On average you need to double your power input in watts to lift your speed from 32km/h to 42km/h! TT bikes exist to reduce your frontal area and improve your aerodynamic shape. They aren't made to be comfortable, and rarely are. But if you intend to ride against the clock in either a triathlon or time trials, you may well find yourself climbing aboard one. If you want to ride an aero bike, then a specific bike fit will be necessary. All the rules change and your existing bike fit metrics will be of limited use.

- Mountain bike – although little mentioned in this book, mountain biking is actually one of our favourite ways to ride a bike. On a cross or gravel bike, it's often the journey that's important; the fact that your bike can take you across a variety of terrain. An MTB is for off-road connoisseurs who often have an intrinsic enjoyment of the terrain itself. Long-travel suspension systems, big tyres and high skill levels all determine what's possible. It's one of the best ways to get fit and increase your riding skills, and we always head for the trails once the thermometer dips below three degrees. A gravel or cross bike will take you further, but a well set-up mountain bike will often allow you to explore and enjoy what's right in front of you.

Given my day job, my cognitive bias is that a well-conceived custom frame will serve your long-term interests and help you achieve your cycling goals without disappointment or injury. In our defence, we've spent 20 years helping folk try to extricate themselves from poor bike-to-person relationships. In that sense we're bound to see more riders who are having problems than ones who aren't. But whether you're contemplating a stock bike or a custom one, please remember that your body, under your conscious radar, will always do its best to adapt to the new environment it finds itself in. Many of these adaptions are unhelpful and problematic and can lead to acute chronic problems over time. Your bicycle can be the most freedom-inducing and liberating device that has ever been invented, by harnessing your human potential and redirecting it into kinetic circular drive. But sometimes something gets lost in translation and you may not realise until further down the road. The skill here is to allow the heart its fullest expression – buying a new bike is joyful. But allow your head to have the last word. If you can.

7

FOOD FOR SPORT

A professional grand tour is a travelling circus. A couple of hundred protected souls, self-selected by extreme one-in-a-million genetics and an unhealthy attitude towards pain – their own and that of their fellow competitors. They are supported by hives of worker bees – mechanics, soigneurs, doctors, directeurs sportifs, and so on. As bike fitters we would join the circus as and when we were needed (and then leave again). We'd be parachuted into a hotel in Belgium or Yorkshire armed with a list of ailments that needed closing off – physically, but often mentally; physical issues are emotionally draining when your body's performance is your living. It always struck us as ironic that riders who could attack some of the most extreme roads in the world, often lined with screaming fans, desperate for blood and glory, functioned in a hermetically sealed bubble of in loco parentis pastoral protection when they were off the bike. And the one thing they loved above everything else was the food that they ate. Most top teams take their own chef out on the road, who sources the freshest food from local markets, while the riders are racing or sleeping. We could be in superb hotels known for their cuisine, with lauded chefs, but the riders only ever ate what their personal chef prepared for them. Only the riders would eat the food prepared by their chef – not even the team owner or directeur sportif was ever allowed to touch the food that was prepared for the riders. Taking a rider's bike for a spin round the block was way less of a crime than tucking into Fabian Cancellara's raisin-soaked bircher muesli. Which was what I was happily doing when the big man himself moved smoothly alongside me, in order to quietly put me straight. Many famous riders aren't in the least bit intimidating – they love riding their bikes and the feeling it gives them. They are just regular guys who happen to be very good at racing. Fabian was also very good at riding his bike, but he was also an effortlessly charismatic perfectionist leader. And at that moment, I, the lowest rung on the circus ladder, stood between him and his breakfast, the opening portion of the maybe 7000 calories that he would need to eat that day to get around the stage. I felt a little like a scavenging fox between a lion and his kill. I duly skulked off, back to the crunchy nut cornflakes. Tour riders march on their stomachs. Nothing is given more priority in the circus than the food they eat. How was I to know?

Middle-aged athletes probably also march on their stomachs, but not so much is known about our nutritional requirements and how they may change over time as we continue to exercise for performance gain, and not just maintenance of fitness.

It's a state of affairs I have become quite used to for almost every topic covered in this book. Kathryn Brown, British Cycling, English Institute of Sport, Senior Performance Nutritionist, says: 'I don't think there's a whole heap of research in masters' nutrition from the performance perspective.'

Kathryn Brown sounded more surprised than I felt. As I have said before, we're the pioneers and trailblazers and our participation in high level sport, especially cycling, will be prompting research studies into how we're impacted differently to younger athletes for years to come. One of those studies will deal with nutrition. Sports nutrition is a huge subject on its own – I'll not try covering its complexity and subtlety here. I will, however, try to highlight how our nutritional requirements change as we age, especially if we try to maintain or even intensify our athletic function.

Left to its own devices, our muscle mass will peak at around 30, gently ebb away through our 40s, really start to fall away in our 50s and

60s before tumbling away at a truly alarming rate in our 70s and 80s. We learned in chapter 1 that this natural age-related decline, sarcopenia, is the adversary of midlife athletes. But Kathryn Brown introduces a new concept into our understanding of sarcopenia that's not related to strength or power: 'A reduction in muscle mass leads to a reduction in metabolic rate because the muscles are the metabolically active tissue in our bodies. The higher your muscle mass, the higher your resting metabolic rate will be and the easier it will be to stay lean and strong.' If there has ever been a starker example of 'youth being wasted on the young', then I have never heard it.

This means that as we get older and lose muscle our metabolic requirements decline and therefore our energy intake should decline. Actually, the 'right' to eat is probably the one thing that would motivate me to get to the gym.

The positive interpretations of Kathryn Brown's insight into muscle as metabolically active tissues are, firstly, that she's singing loudly and in tune with the rest of the clinical choir in this book – midlife athletes need to incorporate resistance training into their diet, in a way they may not have needed in their 20s and 30s. And secondly, that older athletes need to develop a nutrition strategy to mitigate against the worst effects of sarcopenia, while at the same time managing their weight. A net reduction in muscle mass would suggest that we need to reduce our energy intake because we now have a corresponding decrease in our metabolic rates. The middle-age spread isn't a cliché, it's a very real mismatch between calorie intake and expenditure.

Dropping out a session of road miles once or twice a week in favour of structured resistance training could, in theory, be better for our overall health and performance in terms of weight management, bone density, muscle preservation and even neural plasticity and cognition. It's ironic that younger riders arguably need to go to the gym and do less weight training than their parents, but all the experts and clinicians I spoke to agreed on this one reality.

Beyond the age of 50, the way we metabolise food and store energy as carbohydrate and fat alters as we become less insulin-sensitive over time – but even that in itself can be somewhat positively influenced by training. So it's important to keep the oxidative, low-intensity road sessions as well as the resistance training sessions, because this will help the body learn to use fat stores as a fuel source as well as boost the mitochondria within the muscles.

Kathryn Brown suggests that midlife athletes have higher protein requirements than younger ones due to 'anabolic resistance', which is a declining ability to use the amino acids from the proteins to synthesise muscle. She says: 'Older athletes just need a bit more protein to stimulate that pathway.'

As a general guideline, the younger athletes that are looked after by British Cycling typically consume 0.3 grams of protein per kilogram of body weight every 3–4 hours. Middle-aged or older athletes should consume a bit more, for example 0.4 grams. This works out at 30–40 grams of protein per meal time, which is more than a younger athlete requires for the same body weight. 30–40 grams is actually quite a lot and equates to five eggs or four cups of milk. Taking in this much protein to supplement your training will need thought if, for example, you are to avoid increasing your red meat consumption. This is a clear change in approach and lifestyle from our younger selves which we could all follow as we age to try managing progressive loss of muscle mass. It does need to be accompanied with structured resistance training.

In terms of the type of proteins that we should consume, there's some evidence to suggest that proteins derived from animal fats tend to be slightly higher quality because they have a proportionally higher 'leucine' content. Leucine is an essential amino acid that acts as a precursor for protein synthesis and muscle growth. Including leucine in our diet is especially important for midlife athletes trying to prevent muscle loss, meaning all of us. Essential amino acids, by the way, are so called because they are the ones that your body cannot make itself.

The kinds of food that are rich in leucine are dairy products such as cheese and eggs, as well as meat and fish. If you don't want to consume animal products, you can meet your leucine requirements from plant-based sources such as quinoa, nuts, peas and soy beans. Kathryn Brown makes the point that if you have a solely plant-based diet it's possible to get all the proteins and amino acids that you need but you'll inevitably have to draw from a greater variety of sources.

For the record – I'm entirely morally inconsistent – I don't eat meat, but I do eat dairy and fish. Essentially I don't eat anything with a face I like. It's a position with a lot of holes. But as a friend of mine once remarked: 'There's no such thing as a safe port in a storm when it comes to vegetarianism.'

Eating dairy products helps with protein and leucine but also helps ensure good stocks of another vital dietary nutrient, our old friend from chapter 2 – calcium. Along with vitamin D, this key nutrient ensures good bone minerality. Kathryn Brown reinforces the point that bone density hits a high-water mark at the age of 30 and then starts to decline. In a perfect world our nutrition and exercise strategy to that point will provide a good foundation for middle age. The only problem is that cycling isn't weight-bearing so leaves many of us exposed to osteopenia and osteoporosis if we don't bring something other than cycling into our exercise landscape and we're not careful with our diet. I'm no longer surprised when an ultra-fit client reports back with a borderline, or even osteoporotic, DEXA score. There's definitely something going on here which will ultimately be revealed with additional research. Incidentally, Kathryn Brown shares the view of Dr Hulse, that vitamin D supplementation is one of the few that may be justified outside of normal healthy food intake. Dietary sources of vitamin D are fairly poor, and in the UK we are in the Northern Hemisphere, where for at least six months of the year, we have very little discernible vitamin D from the sun. Winter supplementation for midlife athletes could also help with muscle preservation, as vitamin D is instrumental in protein synthesis.

Another area of contention in veteran athlete nutrition is specifically related to women, and whether they have different requirements to men, especially around menopause. It's thought that there's a drop-off in both muscle bulk and bone density with declining levels of oestrogen, but we don't yet know how far these can be modified in midlife female athletes with specific strength and conditioning sessions, and supplementation.

Most sports physicians and sports nutritionists have an intrinsic antipathy to supplementation – they rightly prefer us to get the nutrients we need from a diversity of real foods rather than rely on something artificially synthesised and put into a capsule. Vitamin D seems to be a possible exception, but are there any others?

Dr Stephens shares the 'real food' philosophy but does take cod liver oil (so do I, by the way). Kathryn Brown can see the sense in supplementing with omega 3 for midlife athletes if they don't regularly eat oily fish, which is one of the highest density sources. Omega 3 is considered a healthy fat in terms of cardiovascular function and has also been linked in studies to protein synthesis. The versatile omega 3 is also known to have anti-inflammatory effects, which is why I started taking it many years ago after sustaining my back injury. I'm not sure that any supplementation is entirely risk-free, but vitamin D and omega 3 seem to be the least controversial and potentially the most beneficial.

Maybe more controversial is iron supplementation. This is popular with athletes, because of its integral role in the haemoglobin in our blood, which is crucial for transporting oxygenated blood from the lungs to our muscles. An iron deficit is devastating for sportspeople because it generally causes deep exhaustion and poor performance. For those reasons, it's often taken pre-emptively, even when it's not necessary. Aside from being toxic in higher quantities, iron can affect the absorption of other minerals our bodies need. Kathryn Brown thinks that iron supplementation should be taken only if a deficit is identified by way of a clinically led blood test.

We worked extensively a few years ago with an elite female racer, whose performance was inexplicably declining over time. She was a train-a-holic with an unassailable work ethic, as well as being one of the mentally toughest racers that we've ever encountered. So when she started underperforming, it was both mysterious and dramatic – her power numbers dropped through the floor and training became impossible. A blood test revealed a significant iron deficiency, which was corrected and monitored by her doctor over a few months. What caused the deficiency in the first place is also an interesting question but, in the first instance, her power, fatigue and mood remedied rapidly over a few weeks. This was a dream diagnosis for an elite athlete – a testable variable that's found to be lacking, followed by a fast-acting, cheap and reliable treatment plan. This particular athlete was sensible to work through her GP and have the whole process professionally assessed and controlled, as well as a further review to look for the underlying cause.

Another supplement that's almost universally associated with cycling is coffee, or caffeine. Tour de France teams are routinely sponsored by coffee companies and there are multiple espresso bars at the start of every stage. It's been used (and probably abused) by amateur and professional cyclists for over 100 years. No big day in the Alps, Pyrenees or Dolomites would ever be quite the same without strategic coffee stops. And for good reason – there's convincing research evidence to show that caffeine does improve both sprint and endurance performance on the bike. So it seems that we get a very real jolt of focus and energy after a double espresso at the base of the Col du Galibier. What's not as well known is that the amount of caffeine required to elicit a tangible performance benefit is actually comparatively low. Kathryn Brown says: 'Research suggests that the optimal dose is 1–3mg per kilogram of body weight, which roughly correlates to only one cup of coffee.'

At the other end of the substance spectrum, alcohol has no palpable performance or health advantage at all. Kathryn, who works with younger elite athletes, says they generally eschew alcohol because it 'impairs post-training recovery, compromises the immune system, decreases reaction time and impairs cognitive performance.'

It's a strange but widespread phenomenon that we tend to increase our alcohol consumption as we get older, even as our ability to metabolise it declines. I saw it with my own father: I used to enjoy a glass or two of red wine with him, but he didn't seem to recognise the fact that its effect upon him changed and escalated over time. Or maybe he did, and drank it anyway. As midlife athletes, we at least have to think about our alcohol consumption if we want to optimise both health and performance, even if we then choose to ignore it and not modify our behaviour in any way. It doesn't help anyone that the tabloid consensus over alcohol relentlessly flip-flops from one week to the next. One week the papers are screaming how Brits are all drinking too much, wrecking our physical and mental health. And the next week there will be an article proclaiming that moderate drinking promotes cardiovascular or cognitive health and well-being. A more cynical person might suspect that the drink lobby is in one corner and newspapers are in the other, selling themselves via lowbrow headlines, with the public left standing in the middle, puzzled. Whatever strategy with alcohol you ultimately adopt, remember that professional cyclists tend heavily towards the abstemious, precisely because it adversely affects their performance on the bike. I repeat here the suggestion that you moderate, or even stop, your alcohol intake around training and event participation to maximise your long-term health and performance. Having an alcohol strategy makes sense as we get older and at the same time are trying to coax more performance from our bodies.

If we do decide to keep consuming alcohol as we train and compete, Kathryn Brown has one more thought for us – there's some evidence to suggest that drinking cherry juice in the evening can boost our melatonin levels and thereby help us surrender to a restful sleep and resist waking up at three in the morning.

To recap, here are nine simple rules, for food for sport:

1   A nutrition strategy for older athletes should take into account age-related muscle loss and anabolic resistance – we should proportionally increase our protein intake as we age.

2   Muscles are our metabolically active tissue – we need to do all we can to preserve them.

3   Our resting metabolic rate declines as we age. We can offset this by weight training and increasing protein consumption in our diet. But we may still need to eat less overall to restore our resting metabolic rate (RMR) energy balance.

4   We should ideally get all the nutrients and minerals we need from real food. It's the safest and healthiest way to get all of our requirements.

5   Vitamin D is one possible exception to the supplementation rule, as we may not get enough from natural sunlight and food in more northerly climes. It has such a pivotal role in many of our body's key processes that supplementation may be justified. Overdosing is rare because the body will self-regulate absorption through the skin if adequate stores are already provisioned.

6   There's evidence that omega 3 has a role in promoting cardio-vascular health and reducing inflammation in the body.

7   Caffeine, in low-to-moderate doses, can increase sprint and endurance performance.

8   Ethanol (alcohol) inhibits performance and recovery to an increasing degree as we age. It also appears to affect heart rhythms, even in low qualities.

9   If it all gets too much, cherry juice will put us to sleep.

Eat your age

There's a little ritual that's often played out in Cyclefit sessions. It's the point where we ask a middle-aged athlete their weight. The reply is often emotionally loaded – many of us are positively or negatively invested in our weight. The reply often goes something like this: '75kg. I have been since I was 19 years old.' It invites so much deconstruction:

- You're not 19 any more.
- You may well be the same weight as you always were but you're almost certainly not the same fat-to-lean-muscle-mass composition, due to anabolic resistance.
- Your cells regenerate every seven to 10 years. You're constantly changing, so your 19-year-old self has long gone.
- A 55-year-old isn't merely a young person who became old.

It's pure denial to try pretending we're the same and unchanging. It's as irrational as trying to squeeze into the Levi 501s that I used to wear 30 years ago and then convincing myself that I am neither an eyesore nor in a huge amount of discomfort.

Being a successful midlife athlete isn't about living life as if you were half your age (or less). It's about gracefully and rationally accepting the arc of life, with all of its challenges, and from that point setting strategies, where you can, which will best ameliorate the effects of ageing on both health and performance. Our Peter Pan clients can be quite hard to work with; the body got old but the mind refused to accept it. They are the ones I worry about most – they remind me of Icarus, flying too close to the sun because they refuse to become wise as they get old. We tend to see them on the almost inevitable downslope when they are either overtrained, chronically injured, overtired or their nutrition is a mess. They have eaten the candle after burning it at both ends. We thoroughly support the quest to be immoderate in terms of our exercise aspiration and application as we get older. But there is no place for delusion here. We are not physically young and therefore almost certainly cannot take performance and health for granted as we once maybe could. It is possible to achieve remarkable things on our bike as we age, but this is almost always within the context of better preparation, planning and information.

Nutrition is a neat microcosm of the effects of ageing and shows how we should both expect and embrace change. Where you can emulate your younger self is in your mental agility to accept transformation. If you want your performance curve to keep ticking up with the years, you should modify your diet or even accept that you can no longer metabolise alcohol as efficiently as you used to and still train the next day. It may be that you should think about your meat consumption habits and reduce those elements that are known to be nutritionally poor and which may have deleterious effects on your health, such as sausages, burgers and bacon. Eat much less meat but maximise your nutritional dividend by making sure it's organic and high in lean protein. Getting old and getting faster is inevitably about making more, and better, choices than when we were younger, and a huge component of that is what we choose to consume.

8

THE MINDFUL CYCLIST

This chapter was one of the last to be formulated and written. The wellspring was the sum of all of the interviews and correspondence that I had with Dr Parry-Williams when I was researching the book. I was always keen to cut to the heart of the matter, looking for simplistic, statistically significant conclusions and trends that could act as informed breadcrumb trails, which we could all follow to maximise performance while at the same time minimising risk of harm. Dr Parry-Williams was always a patient and a wonderful tutor, explaining the complexity of human heart activity as we exercised hard and packed on the years. I lost count of the number times she used the words 'We just don't know yet, Phil' in response to my impatient request for binary clarification.

But I always got the impression that along with not knowing, Dr Parry-Williams did have some subjective theories about how veteran athletes – and let's be honest here, mostly men – could positively effect their physical and mental health and the connection between the two. This chapter could also be called 'What about the rest of it?' because most of the iceberg lurks beneath the surface and can't be observed or necessarily measured. Bikes, training, food, injuries, heart rate and even heart attacks can all be assessed and physically metricated. But there's another layer here. A foundational substrate that underpins our physical, mental and emotional well-being. It is the 'anything else' that glues us together as functioning people and, by extension, athletes. The 'mindful cyclist' is one who takes care of their whole self and in doing so makes themselves a faster cyclist and almost certainly a better parent and partner.

If you've made it this far through the book you'll know that cycling alone isn't enough to ensure general health, or indeed maximum performance, as we progressively age. The fact that there are no 50-year-old Moto GP racers, boxers or even chess champions demonstrates that we're swimming gallantly against the genetic tide. But the big swim is incredibly worthwhile – the physical, cognitive and emotional benefits of staying match fit as we get older are profound and precious.

At every turn, new research is being conducted around veteran and masters athletic performance. Fascinatingly, recent studies have suggested that the reason chess champions are comparatively young (20–30 years old) is because 'fluid' intelligence peaks in our early 20s. Fluid intelligence is thought to be responsible for inductive reasoning, spatial awareness and reaction time – all good attributes for abstract puzzle-solving like chess. Inductive reasoning may be a young person's game because it necessarily utilises some calculation of probability or risk: 'It walks like a duck, quacks like a duck – it's probably a duck.' By contrast, deductive reasoning follows prescriptive logic – 'All men are mortal, Aristotle is a man, Aristotle is mortal.' Conversely, crystallised intelligence – responsible for deduction, knowledge and application of practical experience – is relatively stable until we're in our mid-60s. One of the factors that may lead to a decline in fluid intelligence is a simple lack of repeated practice. That's to say, we stop playing chess or otherwise forcing our brains to make these fast synapse connections. Or possibly we just become more cautious as we get older and therefore increasingly uncomfortable with the risks and assertions of inductive reasoning?

I contend that riding a bike fast down a mountain, or holding your position in a fast-moving peloton, is three-dimensional chess played at warp speed. So, it must be superb for maintaining or increasing fluid intelligence. You don't know what is around the corner, or what the other riders are going to do, so you have to make some reasonable assumptions about what is going to happen in a fast-moving dynamic scenario – pure inductive reasoning, fluid intelligence training. If this book were being written in 2050 and not 2020, there would be far fewer unknowns. We're the pathfinders, the first generation to eschew getting old, fat, and pulling out the all-you-can-eat cruise brochures in sufficient numbers to be statistically interesting to medical and sports science. People certainly did ride their bikes up and down mountains when they were 55 in previous decades, but they were outliers. Now, however, it may still be commendable and laudable to ride your bike up a few alpine climbs, but it is happily far from remarkable. That genie is out of the lamp and is not going back in. Expect many more 50- and 60-year-olds to have a physical form that resembles and performs much closer to their 30-year-old selves than their parents at the same age. Our expectation around ageing is shifting. We're fully aware of our evolutionary irrelevance and in no denial at all about the process of senescence, but we're also capable and willing to use the stimulus effects of exercise to mitigate the effects of ageing where we can. This isn't some Peter Pan syndrome – it's level-headed intrinsic enjoyment of hard exercise for its own sake, while at the same time increasing long-term mental and physical function.

The fact remains, however, that to perform at a higher level as we grow older requires us to leave no stone unturned and to consider every issue – sleep, alcohol, stress levels, how much coffee we drink, as well as what we eat, how, or even if we train. Every assumption has to be challenged and held up to the light.

Doing more

Simply riding your bike and undertaking no other exercise is probably a poor strategy, especially if most of your riding is inside rather than outside – the former could encourage dehydration, overexertion and limited cognitive engagement in terms of terrain change and machine control. Riding indoors will almost certainly not positively contribute to maintaining your fluid intelligence. But even if you ride outside for most of your training, there are almost certainly a few better strategies to optimise your physical, mental and emotional well-being. We know that we should start resistance training to offset both muscle and bone mineral loss. There are eminent sports physiologists (quoted in this book), who believe, with some evidence, that heavy resistance training will increase our muscle (and bone) density, even if those specific muscles aren't being worked. This means that heavy upper body weights will help muscle fibre maintenance and bone density in our legs. If we can't countenance weights (and I find this one difficult), we could schedule a couple of demanding Ashtanga yoga classes per week, or think about a complimentary sport that involves standing up, balancing, and developing trunk and back strength – I've already suggested paddleboarding. Whatever it is you choose, you have to do something in addition to cycling – it will keep you fresh, help your fluid intelligence, stop you overtraining on the bike and increase your neural plasticity. It will help keep you young in mind and body. This may take some planning and logistics, but it's important to find a physical activity outside cycling that pushes your mind and body in a different dimension. Cycling has been fortunate enough to be a migration destination from other high-impact sports because it's inherently kind to our joints and tendons, but it's not enough on its own as we become midlife athletes.

Emotional equilibrium

Chapter 3 touched on the role of the autonomic nervous system (ANS) as a possible contributor to systemic inflammation and stress. Both inflammation and stress are needed and can be positive in the right context – training provides a stimulus of both, which the body overcomes to strengthen and rebuild itself. But too much stress and spending too long in a state of sympathetic 'fight or flight' arousal is fatiguing and quite possibly systemically inflammatory. We wondered if there was a sex disparity in the way that men and women deal with inflammation and their associated health outcomes. Dr Parry-Williams theorises outside of her cardiologist role: 'Maybe there's something about modern society and the conditions imposed upon men that prevents them from expressing their emotions, resulting in retained stress. There's a good reason why women who love to sit and chat and put the world to rights also get depressed, but also have lower suicide rates and don't get coronary heart disease!'

I put a similar point to Philip Goulder, Professor of Immunology at Oxford University, that there may be a difference in the way we manage our lives, stress and inflammation, and that this is associated with sex. He makes the point that in an evolutionary sense males and females of all species are designed quite differently, so in the ancestral environment the success of males would be largely judged on how many offspring they had. Males evolved to compete and breed for a relatively short amount of time. Evolution, however, advanced females with a superior immune system (two X chromosomes), and therefore a longer and more healthy life. As Professor Goulder notes: 'So, testosterone makes big muscles at the expense of investment in the immune response. Females need to invest more in the quality of their offspring, and hence in themselves.'

The ANS evolved to deal with this ancestral environment where most of the time could be spent in a parasympathetic state, punctuated by the occasional leopard or rival village attack that would provoke a huge jolt of adrenaline and entry into a sympathetic state. There aren't many situations in modern society when the sympathetic state is useful or advantageous. But we have the hardware and it's attenuated to perceive risk or threat, whether it's rational or not (almost always not). And it seems plausible that women are much better equipped at dealing with managing stress and autonomic nervous system equilibrium than men. A possible consequence may be that female veteran athletes aren't adversely affected by coronary heart disease or arrhythmias that are presumed in many cases by cardiologists to have an antecedent in inflammation.

Training, and especially intense interval training, or competition on the bike can trigger a sympathetically activated state in both males and females – your autonomic nervous system finds it difficult to distinguish between a mortal attack on your being and an adrenaline spike from a criterium. Add in a pile of deadline stress at work, three coffees and a lack of sleep, and you'll be ratcheting up your sympathetic nervous system – possibly without a well-rehearsed and easily accessed ladder to climb down.

Being a mindful cyclist, then, involves implementing some anti-inflammatory or parasympathetic strategies to reduce systemic stress. This could involve half a bottle of red wine of an evening (more on that later) or, more sustainably, perhaps yoga or regular meditation. Both of the latter have been shown to be a very effective method of invoking the slow-acting parasympathetic nervous system (PSNS) in response to a sympathetic nervous system (SNS) alarm call. Incidentally, the yoga should be the slower, flowing vinyasa type of class, where there's an emphasis on moving between poses using your breath. Ashtanga yoga, which is more strenuous, could arguably have the opposite effect.

Essentially, we're looking for any coping strategy that will help us slow down and take a breath – literally and metaphorically. In its simplest form it can be just focussing on your breathing, making sure that you breathe out longer than you breathe in; and this is the easiest and most convenient way to invoke your PSNS if you feel yourself getting wound up. Slightly more structured is the square breathing we saw in chapter 3. In fact, ICU Consultant Dr Mandeville (we met him earlier, if you remember, in distress after a strenuous indoor cycling session) routinely uses square breathing before he starts any complex procedure or operation. It helps him slow down, relax and focus by consciously moving himself into a parasympathetic state.

Moving towards a parasympathetic state will move you from fight or flight into rest and digest equilibrium – a much healthier and happier place to live most of the time. Remember that you can't properly recover from a training session unless you enter a parasympathetic state.

If we're going to push our bodies physically, on and off the bike, we'll also need to rethink how we help the recovery and supercompensation process by making sure we're relaxed. But how do you know if you're the kind of person who tends to hang out in state of sympathetic arousal? You probably have an innate sense of this yourself – but for the sake of clarity, here are some other clues:

- Do you struggle to relax?
- Do you find it hard to meet all your deadlines?
- Are you poor at multitasking?
- Do have a tendency to live life at a fast pace?
- Do you struggle to juggle all of your responsibilities?
- Do you use coffee and alcohol as stimulants and relaxants?
- Do you have inconsistent sleep patterns?

My hand was up for most of those, by the way. This turbocharged living strategy is unlikely to be the most effective in the Indian summer of our competitive careers. We therefore need an effective way to track and, if necessary, reset our ANS, to protect us from damaging stress and possible inflammation as we simultaneously train and age.

Heart rate variability (HRV)

Athletes can't rely on purely tracking heart rate to see how sympathetically activated they are, because many have low resting heart rates that can somewhat mask the symptoms. A better guide to both autonomic function and your state of recovery is to use HRV. We may think of our hearts banging away like a drum machine, keeping predictable time based on exercise/stimulus inputs. We even use the language of beats per minute (bpm) to describe our heart's rhythm, as if it were a dance track. But while drum machines are designed to thud away at a totally uniform and predictable tempo, our hearts are not. We may be beating at an average of 90bpm, but the gaps between successive beats will be subtly different. Counter-intuitively, the greater the fluctuation between the beats, the more likely you are to be in a parasympathetic phase – that is to say, relaxed and recovered. A low heart rate variability between the beats suggests that the sympathetic nervous system is dominant and that you may well be stressed, and most likely require additional rest and recovery before embarking on another training session. Knowing your HRV will also allow you to actively intervene against low variability – do some meditation, focus your breathing or get some sleep. It's a clear signal that you need to slow everything down to bring yourself back into healthy equilibrium. So a high degree of HRV is desirable because it shows an elasticity of response in the heart to physiological or emotional shifts. A low variation, by contrast, signifies the heart response to stimulus is dulled and sluggish – this wouldn't be a good moment to put your cardiovascular system under load by going out training.

Good HRV has also been shown to be well correlated with high levels of cognitive function and, correspondingly, low HRV values show an impairment in this regard. We all know how it feels to try to conduct high-level thinking or make an important decision when we're tired and stressed. Knowing our HRV as midlife cyclists seems essential if we're going to avoid the pitfalls of overtraining and declining performance. Twenty-five years ago, we used to record our waking resting pulse to establish how fatigued we were and, as a consequence, how hard we should train on that day. My own deflection point was around 50bpm. Anything below 50bpm and I considered myself green to go, anything north of 55 was my signal to avoid training and rest. The numbers in between were harder to interpret, but I would probably ride gently if my resting pulse were between 50 and 55bpm. HRV is a much more sophisticated and informative way of making training decisions.

I may be a barefoot cyclist by instinct but I'm also rational. Even I can see that HRV is a powerful tool for measuring and ultimately modifying ANS imbalance, which is umbilically linked to mental and physical well-being. Moreover, this isn't homeopathy or pseudo-science – HRV's application in sports science and mainstream medicine is widespread and it's even used in hospitals to predict mortality risk in patients who have had a heart attack. As we get older and try to chase the cycling dream upstream against the natural flow of the ageing process, it makes no sense to focus on FTP as our preferred metric unless we're also equally fixated by the underlying foundation measurement of our physical and mental health – HRV. You can easily track HRV using your heart monitor chest strap and downloading one of the many apps out there. There are a couple that use the light from your smartphone to trace and record HRV so you don't have to use the chest strap. Even easier is a smart watch that will accurately track HRV all the time so you can understand your own trends and rhythms. You'll see as you exercise that your HRV will reduce and then increase as you rest and recover. If it doesn't, then you know right away to back off and add in more recovery time.

Training hard is innately acutely (in the moment) inflammatory and chronically (over time) anti-inflammatory. It's our responsibility to manage the twin inputs of exercise and recovery to manage these levels of inflammation and fatigue. There's just something about cyclists – they've never been very good at managing this. I asked Dr Baker how many of his amateur clients were overtraining when they were first referred to him and he said: "Honestly, Phil, almost all of them. We can't go forwards until we take a step back. They almost all go on a diet of oxidative base, so they can build up and become faster again.'

It appears that we all seem to train ourselves to exhaustion, and it doesn't get better as we age – we just don't seem to get any wiser. With running, it's literally very hard to put one foot in front of the other and run if you're chronically fatigued, but somehow you can always clamber aboard a bike, plonk yourself on the saddle and grind out another 50km.

Running is so ballistic and high-loading that the inherent trauma is brought into sharp focus if you try to run when you're tired or generally feeling below par. I suggest that midlife athletes allow HRV to be their guide here again, to become more attenuated to our physical and emotional needs. There's zero positive training effect in going out riding if you're recovering from a virus or have just done too much. If you do record a low HRV number, maybe the most pragmatic strategy for long-term health and performance would be: rest, meditation and gentle breathing yoga class until your HRV rises back to normal again.

And there seems to be some sexual dimorphism here. Male veteran athletes are most at risk from cardiac complications, have weaker immune systems, and yet are still more likely to indulge in less pragmatic lifestyles and training choices. I asked Professor Goulder about this. He said: 'I agree that males and females of all species are designed differently. The ultimate cause of sexual selection is the different size of the gametes and from this differences in appearance, behaviour and the immune system are selected in males and females of the same species. It's a massive topic . . . the consequence is that males tend to live shorter lives.'

It's not only that males are quite possibly genetically predisposed to have weaker immune systems but that male 'behaviour' also plays a huge role. At the time of writing we're going through the Covid-19 crisis – I sincerely hope that as you read this it's just a distant memory. The early signs are that men are twice as likely, maybe even more, than women to die of this virus. There may be some sociological and behavioural explanations but much of the disparity is probably driven by genetics. And yet we're also less likely to try to understand our inherent frailties and vulnerabilities.

Dr Parry-Williams steps out of her cardiologist role for a moment to express her personal opinion on the subject. 'I think women athletes benefit hormonally but are also more self-expressed and therefore more aware, and therefore have more ability to transform difficult emotions into positive ones, and also get support. Being listened to is therapeutic in itself, hence why we maybe communicate more.'

It's irrational for male veteran athletes to acknowledge the ageing process and try to ameliorate the worst effects with hard training on the one hand and, on the other, to fail to acknowledge that we're also susceptible to poor health outcomes due to our gender, genetics and embedded behaviours, and not want to counteract that as well. We just can't afford to selectively pick the bits of science and evidence that we like and ignore the bits we don't. It negatively influences both our well-being and our performance on the bike. So we're happy to obsess about FTP and work hard to increase that by five watts, not so willing to look at our levels of accumulated stress, inflammation, and fatigue. I started going to a few yoga classes (the easier vinyasa ones) with my wife, and ususally there was myself and sometimes one other man in a room of 30 women. What's going on with men? What are we missing?

HRV may have the potential to get through to the minds of male masters cyclists because it is scientifically uncontested and reduces complex, bottled-up emotions to a number that can be digested, comprehended and, crucially, acted upon. I realise that these are not easy issues. But we have to make sure we are wise before we are old, and taking these little practical steps can be a commitment to that. Dr Parry-Williams again: 'Heart rate variability is a marker of autonomic function – athletes are using it a lot now for recovery from training, meaning that if their heart rate variability isn't restored then it's a sign they haven't physically recovered, so athletes employ HRV to prevent overtraining.'

The myth of periodisation – confronting an inconvenient truth

The importance and possible ramifications of our emotional state, and especially our background stress levels, on training and performance were highlighted by a strength and conditioning coach, John Kiely. In his radical paper, Kiely challenges the assertion that improvements in fitness based on physical exercise are predictable, and that these improvements are only directed and determined by the physical stress of the training. Or to put it another way, Kiely fundamentally questions the largely unexamined, seven-decade assertion that 'training stress directly regulates the magnitude of subsequent "fitness" adaptations.'

Kiely even attempts to explain why the current periodisation model of training is simplistically based on very old research into the science of stress, which may have seemed rational and consistent in the 1920s, but could now do with a refresh. Kiely even cites the same example of the QWERTY keyboard and notion of 'path dependence' that I used in chapter 2. As a quick refresh, path dependence is the concept that an idea gets somehow preserved in aspic and then thrown forwards into the future, largely unchallenged, into an era that would reject it if it cared to question its modern application. We looked at the bicycle and the QWERTY keyboard – and now the entire model of periodised training is coming under scrutiny!

Most sports science, especially coaching and periodised training, stands on the unwilling shoulders of endocrinologist Hans Selye, and his research into how organisms react to stress, which he called general adaption syndrome (GAS). Selye concluded that reactions to stress were predictable and measurable – and the concept and language was wholeheartedly commandeered by coaches and sports scientists. Kiely eloquently and plausibly challenges the limits of the periodisation model and its 'implicit assumption that mechanical loading parameters directly dictate biological training adaptations.'

Kiely contends that training and athletic performance shouldn't be viewed as abstract or distinct from our psychological and emotional state. And that our stress, happiness, tiredness and emotional balance should be perceived as being important variables, which will directly affect the outcome of every exercise session and our overall performance and health.

He's obviously right – as you read the paper it's impossible not to share his epiphany – even before he presents the metadata around athlete injury and performance related to stress. His conclusions are arguably even more important for midlife athletes – we're inherently more fragile than we were in our 20s and invariably carrying more responsibility and, with it, stress. 'Mounting evidence illustrates that excessively accumulating multi-source stress variously down-regulates the immune system, motor coordination, cognition, mood, metabolism, and hormonal health; thereby dampening positive adaptation, diminishing athletic performance, elevating injury risk, and compromising recovery and recuperation.'

It's so much easier to measure power, speed, weight, time and heart rate than it is stress, happiness, worry and depression. And it may therefore be natural for us to gravitate towards numerical variables rather than more nebulous emotional ones, however important they are.

In some ways Kiely's ideas are a little Foucauldian (see chapter 4) in the sense that he proposes that there should be room for introspection, negotiation and an honest appraisal of how one feels physically and emotionally, in relation to a training regime. A Foucauldian 'do what you feel' approach presupposes that you know what you feel, which itself presumes you're in the habit of asking yourself the question 'How do I feel?' In this particular regard, Kiely also discusses the idea that HRV is a 'biologically oriented indicator of current stress conditions' in the context of ANS function.

It cannot be an accident that there are many forces converging on the mind–body connection when it comes to training, and especially midlife exceptionalism. Dr Parry-Williams, John Kiely and Dr Hulse all seem to be of one mind – that what's happening emotionally is as important as what's happening physically for our long-term fitness and health.

243

The next time you're about to do your fourth indoor FTP session of the week, ask yourself these questions: Am I tired? Am I bored? Do I feel stressed? Is this what I need to do? Will this help my long-term goals? Will this help my general health and well-being? If it's yes to all of the above, then crack on. If a couple of noes creep in, then maybe step back and reappraise for a moment.

Abstinence makes the heart grow stronger

This may well be one of the more controversial sections of the book. Wine seems to be as ready an accompaniment to cycling as strong coffee. Well, it was for me. I remember riding with some Italian friends the day before participating in the colossal Pinarello Gran Fondo event, in the Veneto area of northern Italy. We stopped at several farms as we traversed the bean-shaped Montello. Every farmer bought out a jug of prosecco, made using grapes grown on their own land. We sat on trestles and drank the prosecco as a refreshing mid-morning tonic. Some of the farms served salty parma ham and cheese, and local 'mintele' crackers to complement the light acidity of their sparkling wine. Even so, at the last farm, I was relieved to see my wife and our host's wife, Bruna, in a car. There's no way I could have safely contemplated another farm courtyard and flagon of local prosecco, however light and bubbly it was. Therefore, a sinner like me would do better being the last to proselytise about mixing alcohol and cycling – before, after, and, in this exceptional case, during.

But there are a few problems connected to being mindful about the timing and extent of our alcohol intake as veteran athletes. Just as our body's relationship to training and recovering evolves as we age, so does our relationship with alcohol and our ability to metabolise it. Alcohol (or ethanol) is thought to be good in very small quantities for general health and the cardiovascular system, under the old principle that 'a little bit of poison does you good.' There is some research to support the role of the polyphenols in red wine and a decrease in exposure to Type 2 diabetes and heart disease. The problem is that the amounts are tiny – under a glass of wine for men, per day, and half a glass for women, which further reduces the older we get. But how can you possibly know that your alcohol intake has any benefit for you as an individual? This will vary from person to person. Personally, I wonder if the studies that have determined ethanol to be beneficial in small quantities have screened for all the confounding variables. Although alcohol is actually bad for us, is its poisonous nature offset by the role it plays in positive socialisation and helping some people to relax? And if alcohol really did have discernible physiological benefits for our heart or cognitive health, would we not have found a way by now to isolate the active compound and put it in a tablet?

As we age we know that we tend to lose muscle bulk (but not after reading this book, of course) and gain fat stores (ditto), both of which result in ethanol having a greater toxic reaction within our bodies, and then being also harder to clear. In part this is because we're generally more hydrated when we're younger – muscles hold more water than fat. Similarly the enzymes in our livers struggle to retain the same effectiveness in clearing ethanol out of our system. Does anyone else find that hangovers seem to get worse as you get older, even when you consume the same number of units as before? 'Alcohol is more toxic in the ageing organism because of changes in its metabolism, distribution and elimination' say Meier and Seitz in their paper 'Age, alcohol metabolism and liver disease'.

But why is this important if we're trying to balance midlife performance on the bike with a midlife proclivity for fine red wine? Kathryn Brown provides a subtle clue from a performance perspective: 'Alcohol isn't essential in someone's diet. In an elite athlete alcohol could impair recovery post-training, compromise the immune system, negatively affect sleep quality and possibly decrease cognitive performance.' For these reasons elite athletes tend not to drink at all despite being better protected against the effects of alcohol by their increased muscularity and youth.

Moreover, alcohol is regarded by the body as a pure toxin and is obligated to deal with it as an immediate priority. This changes our metabolism from the very first glass. Kathryn Brown again: 'Alcohol can reduce fat oxidisation, as you tend to metabolise alcohol first, which is why people with a really high alcohol intake can see an increase in both body weight and body fat.' Well, that doesn't sound ideal for a midlife cyclist.

We also learned in chapter 3 that alcohol can play a contributory role in provoking heart arrythmias, and especially atrial fibrillation (AF). And men are five times more likely to suffer from AF than women. Men have to face facts. They're just not designed as well as women – which possibly explains why we drink in the first place.

The final reason that we may want to ameliorate our alcohol intake if we are in a training block, building to an event, is because of its effect on sleep. When we discussed the stages of training – stimulus, recovery and supercompensation – the 'recovery' phase is really code for sleep. Sleeping is our way of recovering from overexertion. We're just not equipped to recover or enter supercompensation without an abundance of good quality slumber.

REM rebound

Not a Michael Stipe tribute act, but the likely corollary of drinking before we go to bed. Although alcohol pushes us gratifyingly quickly off our conscious ledge into a deep bear-snoring sleep, it then interrupts our regular sleep architecture, causing us to rebound out of the rapid eye movement (REM) phase back into non-REM sleep patterning. REM sleep occupies about one quarter of our total night's sleep – maybe two hours on average. But even though we sleep less as we get older, our total REM burden per night does not vary substantially, so we spend comparatively more time in REM than we did in our 20s and 30s. REM is the phase of sleep where we dream most intensely and yet physically we're at our most incapacitated, as our skeletal muscles lose their tonicity and function. Although REM isn't fully understood, it's thought to be pivotal in both physical and mental recuperation – but it's a physiological and biological requirement that alcohol disrupts. We'll probably wake less rested, less recovered and definitely more grumpy.

I'm not advocating giving up alcohol altogether – it has a potentially powerful social cohesion role and is enjoyed for epicurean and aesthetic reasons when shared with loved ones and friends. I'm suggesting, however, that even moderate alcohol intake is probably inconsistent with overall health and performance if you're a midlife athlete who is in structured training, with specific goals in mind. It may be better to set very tight limits while you're in this phase of your life, or even stop altogether until the end of the season. You'll probably perform better, be healthier and recover faster. A great bottle or two of Brunello di Montalcino is a superb way to reward yourself when your season or event is done.

While we're talking about sleep, it should be noted that 'sleep medicine' is one of the areas that professional teams and Olympic squads have concentrated on to increase athlete performance. Sports science, with all its complexity and emerging technology, has yet to find anything that even fractionally helps our recovery as much as our natural desire to shut down for a third of each day. It's truly when most of the good work gets done. Dr Stephens says: 'The one thing I have focussed on more – because I believe the story behind it – is sleep.'

Sleep architecture or 'sleep hygiene' research has identified a couple of other factors that can help sleep quality and quantity. First, make your sleep patterns more regular – go to bed at the same time and wake up at the same time. The second, is to understand that the blue light from LCD screens, such as smartphones and tablets, decreases the production of melatonin, which, as we discussed in chapter 2, is secreted by the pineal gland. Melatonin is gradually released during the evening as a response to decreased ambient light – it builds up in our bodies to prepare us to go to sleep. The blue light from LCD screens interrupts the production of melatonin, and therefore delays or disrupts our normal pattern of getting tired and naturally falling asleep. Dr Hulse recommends quitting all LCD blue lights at least two hours before going to sleep, otherwise 'it will totally wipe out your melatonin production.'

In the world of professional cycling medicine, it's accepted that getting the right amount of sleep is the single greatest recovery factor for an elite athlete and is of far more use than massages, ice baths and supplements. It's been shown that athletes who get less than eight hours sleep per night are 1.7 times more likely to get injured than those who get the full quota. It's no coincidence that Team Sky famously micro-controlled their riders' sleep hygiene by taking their own mattresses and pillows out on the road, and even experimented with taking a motorhome for their designated lead rider. The UCI (them again) considered this such a huge advantage that they quickly banned it. The rider who sleeps the most will necessarily recover the most. The rider who recovers the most has a huge performance advantage. This was the start of the modern medicine revolution that has started to permeate the professional peloton – do the simple things very well. Many of us don't have sufficient 'good quality' sleep and will therefore perform below our full potential and jeopardise our recovery and health.

Dealing with disappointment

Performance doesn't necessarily ratchet up one way – especially as we get older. Injury, overtraining, illness, underperformance, and sometimes even disillusionment, can all potentially get in the way. And it's often the psychological component that's hardest to deal with – the interruption of freedom, brush with mortality, a sense that it will never come back, or never come back the same. In 20 years of working with clients at all levels we've only had a handful of clients who had to give up cycling completely because of injury or illness issues. Now and again we get a client who's seemingly stuck and absolutely nothing is helping. They often feel like they are caught in a spiralling and accelerating wind that is spinning them around from one 'expert' to another. By this point, Jules and I are normally only peripherally involved – our role will be picked up again on the other side of treatment to assess how the client's cycling biomechanics have been affected. It can seem aimless and dispiriting if you're the person with the injury or problem, but remember Dr Parry-Williams' comment: 'There's no purity in medicine.' Things are rarely as binary as we would like.

Our first responsibility as bike fitters, when a client is ill or injured, is to be professional and know when we don't know. We don't and cannot possibly know everything, but we will have a suggestion or two about who does. Secondly, we have a great contacts book full of people who we think can help, no matter what the issue is – and who, importantly, we think are likely to connect with the client as an individual. One of the biggest factors in moving forwards after a setback is the relationship with the people in whom you place your trust. Thirdly, be available in the background, keep the dream alive, reassure the client that we've been through this before and that there will be rides and climbs and great company at the end of the tunnel.

Let's look at some of the things that can go amiss and the likely routes back to full function.

Trauma

Remember Dr Stephens' insight that as midlife cyclists we're trading the occasional 'orthopaedic incident' for greater cardiovascular and cognitive health. It seems like a fair trade when written on a page, especially if you think of all the great adventures to be had on two wheels. But it's called trauma for a reason and is generally to be avoided wherever possible. How can you avoid getting injured?

1   Riding skills. It's quite simply not enough to keep clicking up your FTP. There's no point in tuning the engine if you don't learn the riding skills to go with that increased power. Understand

how to corner, brake and descend safely with confidence. These are techniques to be learned, in the same way that we're not born with the ability to ice-skate or ski. Riding a bike well is balletic – but has to be learned.

2   Try riding off-road in the winter on a mountain or gravel bike and avoid riding too much indoors, as it will not develop any useful skills.

3   Don't ride on the road if the temperature goes below 3 degrees – it could be freezing at the tops of climbs. More accidents happen in cold weather.

4   Choose a bike with disc brakes, as they have more power and a more consistent feel.

5   Use bigger tyres for more grip (and comfort). 25mm in the summer as an absolute minimum, and 28mm or even 32mm in the winter.

6   Make sure your bike fit is optimised. Adapting around a poorly fitting machine can make you less stable and poised, and put your centre of gravity in a less than ideal place.

7   Improve your general body conditioning. If you do fall off, being stronger and more supple could help ameliorate the worst effects. Look at how pros shrug off spills that would have us queuing up in A&E.

So if the worst does happen and you have an accident and pick up an injury, what should you do? Let's split it into three parts – the crash, the treatment and the legacy. During and after the crash itself, don't be brave – go to a hospital if necessary. Call an ambulance if you or others feel it's necessary. Don't delay, you have only one opportunity to be treated as an emergency – the NHS is centred around throwing masses of resources at someone on first urgent contact. If you fall off in the middle of nowhere and hurt yourself, a broken collarbone could soon be the least of your problems as cold and shock set in after the initial adrenaline surge has worn off. So get into the back of that warm ambulance as fast as you can.

In terms of treatment: now you are a crash-test dummy. You have devolved responsibility to someone else – do as you're directed and follow advice. There may be decisions to make, so have someone with you to help make them – leave a collarbone to heal naturally, or move directly to surgery, for example? Listen and ask questions – what's the doctor really advocating here? What would she or he do if it were their own injury? This stage is critical because if you pass up the opportunity for immediate treatment it could be weeks to get to this point again, even if you have private healthcare. You didn't set off from your house with this in mind, and you're bewildered, sitting in hospital in your ripped precious Rapha kit. But try to stay calm and rational – you're safe, you're in good hands, this moment will pass and become history soon enough. Are you maybe sensing that I'm speaking from a wealth of experience here?

What comes after the trauma and the treatment is the legacy – that's where someone like Cyclefit and/or a physical therapist gets involved. You'll heal much faster than a sedentary person – your fitness and conditioning will put you in the fast lane for recovery.

Training hard into middle age and beyond is undoubtedly superb, building a bulwark of resilience for the times when we're physically and mentally tested. ICU Consultant Dr Mandeville explains that critical care and intensive care units all around the UK screen their patients' fitness for medical intervention using cardiopulmonary exercise testing (CPET) for surgical or medical interventions and predicting likely outcomes. It's widely thought that fitness is as good a predictor of clinical outcome as age.

You will therefore probably astound everyone connected to your treatment. But your body will almost certainly be adapting around the injury – it's critical to have your rehab directed and your position and pedalling technique reviewed. This is the moment where we see athletes

251

picking up adapted habits that need to be rapidly understood, explained and compensated for. For example, an elite veteran athlete – Dr Nigel Stephens – falls off in the winter and suffers a serious fracture to his hip. He has emergency surgery and spends a few days in hospital. Nigel is in a hurry and sees us and his treating physical therapist – Alex Fugallo – 10 days after surgery. Luckily Nigel is a cyclist and not a runner. While it will be months before he is advised to return to running, his consultant has directed that cycling is in fact a suitable rehab tool. When we look at Nigel's pedalling 10 days post-surgery, it's understandably dysfunctional. The injured side is guarded and disengaged and the non-injured side has now become overengaged on the recovery stroke, as an unhelpful compensation. This will almost certainly cause pain and possibly injury to the good side and leave the injured side without the loading it needs to recover properly. The direction is to build a new rehab position – shorter cranks, straight bars, flat pedals, higher front end. This prevents the hip angle being closed at the top of the pedal stroke and gives Nigel the correct proprioceptive feedback about how much to load through the injured and good legs respectively. The damaged side will be down on power initially, as expected, but the motor-patterning of the pedal stroke is well-preserved and entirely functional. Now Nigel can work as hard as he likes to offset the effects of muscle atrophy, keep overall fitness and heal the surgery. We slowly modified the position over the next three months in conversation with both Nigel and Alex. Nigel was able to recover his full championship-winning power and fitness in record-breaking time. You can read Nigel's side of the story in his case study (see p. 272).

Injury and illness

I have put these two together because I'm assuming that both start with symptoms which have an unspecified cause – that's to say, not precipitated by trauma. Both illness and injury can be frustrating because there's often a lag between the onset of symptoms and a subsequent diagnosis and treatment path. People understandably get very stressed and even angry because nobody seems to know what's going on, and even less what to do about it, and it's keeping them from what they love doing. Being a cyclist rapidly becomes central to our identity – it's one of the things that we 'are', rather than just 'do'. It doesn't matter if it's a painful knee, heart problems or an in-growing toenail, it's highly significant if it stops us doing what we love and being who we want to be.

I had a serious bike crash in 2011 which resulted in a fractured spine. The injury was wrongly assessed in A&E as being old and I was discharged. After I was sent home the fracture progressed and I could feel the vertebra starting to bulge and pain intensify. A round of consultant appointments, endless MRIs, x-rays and prodding and poking followed over the next year and a half. The potential consequences of the corrective surgery that was now needed were so serious that everyone involved reverted to the mean of doing nothing – albeit with my best interests sincerely at heart. I had missed the vital opportunity in A&E to have stabilisation surgery that day. Endless rounds of physio followed as I diligently pursued the conservative route, which I suspected would be fruitless. Looking back, I realise that I was profoundly depressed – not only because I was in pain and confused, trying to manage my own care, but because I had lost my own sense of myself as a cyclist. Alex Fugallo was steadfast and clear, always rooted in evidence and fact. It was a new injury and it was progressively getting worse; something needed to be done. The first round of spine-fusion surgery failed and left me in a substantially worse condition, both systemically and orthopedically. Nearly six years after the accident I finally walked into corrective surgery with consultant Stewart Tucker. It was to be an all-day affair. The old metalwork was to come out with substantially more metalwork going in, both from the front through the chest and into my spine from the back. Alex Fugallo attended the surgery and was in theatre all day with Mr Tucker. I was helped to my feet the next day and immediately felt different.

Over the next few weeks my rehab progress was profound and rapid. I even suspected that I would, six years on, be able to cycle again. Three years on from the surgery and I'm riding again. I'll always have pain to manage and work around; however, I can enjoy riding and think about setting modest goals. I'm a cyclist. The experience of getting hurt, and the protracted and convoluted route to getting myself fixed, was, in large part, an impetus to write this book – especially this section. I'm not going to pretend that I always believed I would ride again – I didn't. I was in pain and despondent most of the time. It felt bizarre to spend my working days 'fixing' broken cyclists but to be unable to fix myself. The effects of the injury and failed surgery eventually became a physical block to many aspects of work and life. But the point is that it's now in the rear-view mirror – I can ride again and I can function properly. Thinking about that time, I had a lot going for me – a great family and a professional team that had my back, so to speak. This experience speaks to two things – firstly Dr Parry-Williams' point that there's no purity in medicine, even when it's something that can be measured and quantified, such as a fractured vertebra. And secondly, and most importantly, you will come through this. You won't always feel the same as you do now – a universal truism about life as it is about cycling and injuries. We're growing and shedding experiences all the time, like skin. I can remember that I was once in pain and I was despondent, but I can no longer touch the actual pain or hopeless feelings – they have thankfully passed or I left them behind.

As an aside, I have just returned from Dr Hulse's 50th birthday ride, made remarkable by the fact that he's only 14 weeks post triple-bypass surgery after a heart attack (see his case study, p. 268). We rode for 50km in mixed terrain and stopped for a half-time coffee. All seven of us are proclaimed midlife cyclists and were thrilled to be riding by his side. Dave looked the most calm and fittest I have seen him in years. He rode sensibly but strongly at the front of the group for the entire ride. Dave's admirable progress demonstrates a couple of things. Firstly that his decades of cycling fitness put him onto a cardio-rehab superhighway, and that he has, so far, exceeded all of his medical team's expectations of what could be reasonably expected after such major surgery. And secondly, that Dave has shed a huge amount of skin in the whole process. He's more relaxed and physically stronger than he has been in years. He's changed his way of thinking – it wasn't fixed.

Below, I have assembled my best advice for dealing with protracted injury and illness. I should also say that I have clients and friends who are dealing with, or who have dealt with, much worse issues than mine, with more stoicism and wisdom. I'm grateful for all their advice over the years. Sometimes my fitting studio was like the scene below decks in the film *Jaws*, when Richard Dreyfuss and Robert Shaw competitively compare scars! I genuinely never get bored listening to clients' stories. Here are my top tips:

- You'll not always feel like you do now.
- Medicine is rarely as predictable as we would want, so allow for twists and turns.
- Involve your GP and physio. It will almost certainly not be their first rodeo, even if it's yours.
- Stay physically strong – keep exercising as much as you can. If you do have surgery, it will pay dividends in terms of how fast you heal. It'll also help your emotional well-being. Even taking a brisk walk is great – I used to walk as much as I could when I couldn't cycle.
- Dr Hulse says it best: 'If all you have is a hammer, then all you're looking for is a nail.' Surgeons see medical problems through the prism of surgery. Occasionally they are wrong, so get other opinions.

- Become an expert in your medical issue. Older-style surgeons tend to hate this, but open-minded ones like it. It gives them an opportunity to have a deeper and more honest clinical relationship with you, the patient. Great doctors are honest about the fact that they learn from their patients.
- If you're not sure the case has been made for surgery, pull out and go for more conservative treatment.
- If all else has failed and you just have to have surgery, try to mentally prepare by being as positive as possible about that fact and event. There's no point in worrying or becoming anxious about something that's inevitable. Walk in smiling. It does help.
- *Do your prehab!* This is a big one. However hard it is go into surgery, if you're having it, as strong and as fit as you can be. Muscle loss after surgery can be significant.
- Don't skimp on the rehab. This is obvious I know, but get it all in place early so the conveyor belt is ready to run.
- Eat well. Fast healing (like many other things) marches on your stomach. This is especially true after surgery – the quality of what you eat immediately after theatre is key.
- If you do elect for surgery, make sure you see your surgeon post-operation. Not just a registrar, but the actual surgeon who was responsible for what they did in the theatre.
- Be patient – look to those healing milestones, touch them and calmly move forward to the next. Very soon you'll look back and be pleasantly shocked at how far you've travelled.

Losing the love

Impossible right? Cycling is addictive and losing the love is tantamount to blasphemy. Presuming that you're not injured, and therefore pain isn't holding you back, you're almost certainly in a rut. This could be because you're overtrained (see Matt's fascinating overtraining case study, p. 270), or just plain ol' tired and bored.

In any event, the immediate response should be the same. Stop what you're doing – repetition is clearly not working. We hear it from clients all the time – their FTP is going south, despite everything they are doing. Crawling aboard the bike, on the stationary trainer, for one more assault on an abstract number, which has taken on disproportionate importance, is clearly not going to help. You've either reached, or are close to, your theoretical potential, and are now becoming fatigued and stale. If it is the former – congratulations, you are not going to be the next Peter Sagan at the age of 50, and it is better that you come to terms with that now before you pack in your career to join the circus. If it is the latter, it's time to review your goals and reappraise your methodology for achieving them. What would Dr Hulse, Dr Baker and coach Fox say? Most likely they would all prescribe a few days off the bike completely, followed by a few weeks of scaling back the living-by-the-numbers mentality, and just riding to enjoy yourself instead. Maybe grab a mountain bike or gravel bike and head into the woods, or do something totally different – borrow a canoe, dive in a lake, do some orienteering or (my favourite) get lost in a stream or river on a paddleboard. The important thing is to make a change. If you're training for an important event in a structured way, contact someone like Dr Hulse, Dr Baker or coach Fox, who have heard it all before a thousand times. If you have a coach, you can give them some Foucauldian or John Kiely context about mind-body when it comes to training and performance. If they're sensible they will tell you to 'do what you feel' or encourage a deeper conversation about what you're experiencing. You're not simply the net recipient of periodised stress-induced mechanical improvement – you're a highly complex and sentient individual, a tightly wound Gordian knot of biology and psychology. Underperformance and its bedfellow, loss of interest, should trigger a rational review of all the variables that go into making you a happy cyclist.

Your legs don't make you a cyclist anymore than your FTP or the medals and trophies in a cabinet. A cyclist is a person who rides a bike.

A performance cyclist is a person who seeks to ride a bicycle faster or longer, or maybe both. The mindful cyclist is someone who accepts that how you're functioning as a whole person will necessarily impact on how well you perform on a bike. The mindful cyclist comprehends that we're a complex entanglement of physical and mental stimuli, most of which happens under our conscious radar. To be a mindful cyclist requires making new habits and demarcating time to bring our burden of stress, breathing and autonomic state into regular focus. To understand what happens to our equilibrium when we pile up diverse stimulants such as alcohol, caffeine, heavy training and missed sleep. And most importantly, to understand how this all gets magnified when viewed through the prism of our ageing biology.

EPILOGUE

As we mentioned before, the three most liberating words in my profession are 'I don't know.' It helps if you can immediately follow them with 'but I will find out' or even 'but I know someone who does.' But that's not always the case. It's always hard to sit opposite a client who is in pain, injured or struggling to do what they love most and say 'I don't know' in the face of their unfulfilled goals and dreams. Sometimes the three magic words have a calming effect, and sometimes they elicit the opposite response. But at least we've reset the expectations in the room. I'm professional and experienced, and I'll do my very best, but I'm not going to pretend to have all the answers to every single problem. Our minds and bodies are very complex and although we often fall into broad themes and patterns, this isn't always the case. I remember well a young elite athlete who had taken a fall in a race and injured his shoulder. My task was to get him back into a position he could sustain on his bike, pain-free. After a couple of hours, things were not going well, so I sat down with the rider and his mother. It turned out that the poor man was in agony all the time, even as we spoke, and could only function on the strongest opiate-based pain-control.

The cause of his pain had been removed by surgery – there should have been nothing that could sensitise his shoulder to this degree. But 'could' and 'should' mean nothing when someone is in so much pain that it's corroding their daily life, never mind being able to perform on a bicycle. I had nothing to offer, I really didn't know what to do. He needed a neurologist and a specialist in pain control, but he had already seen them, with no improvement. Sometimes there's a huge gap between wanting to help and being able to help. I called the session to an end. Shoulder injuries can be problematic – the shoulder is a joint with a huge range of movement to control, and shoulder pain is anecdotally known to be particularly gruelling. However, this man wasn't following the predicted treatment and rehab pathway, of which I should have been the very last staging post. He was an outlier, and his pain could neither be explained or ameliorated. I don't know what happened to this athlete or whether he was able to resolve his shoulder pain. Add that 'don't know' to the list.

Writing this book has been, in many ways, an exercise in not knowing. And just as with my day job, my first inclination is always to find someone who does know – like a cardiologist, for example. My expectation was that just because I didn't know, someone else would have a deep understanding of how intense and prolonged exertion would impact on an ageing athlete's physiology. This wasn't always the case.

I was lucky to have generous access to two research cardiologists and two front-line treating cardiologists – all connected in some way with midlife cycling. All were disarmingly frank about what is known about intense training into midlife and beyond, and what's still out there to be discovered. There was no pretence, posturing or bluffing from any of them – all were passionate, engaged, caring and insightful. But equally, none pretended to have all the answers. Their haste to say the words 'we just don't know' may be a ground-in professional ethic but they also seemed to revel in the knowledge gaps because the search was still on, the intellectual game still afoot.

When we look back at this book in 20 years time, and I'm almost 80 (busy writing *The Twilight Cyclist*), there'll be far fewer unknowns on the subject of veteran performance cycling. But right now, true to form, we're running ahead of the pack and ahead of the research.

We started in the prologue with the premise that you could stick a pin in almost any date in the last 200,000 years, and the chance of any one of us surviving into our 40s, never mind our 50s, was vanishingly small. Literally only a few decades on from clambering aboard the lifeboat of middle-age survival, we midlife cyclists are setting courses for ambitious destinations. We want fitness levels that in many cases we haven't had since college days, or maybe ever. Many of you reading this will be the fittest you've ever been. It's astounding how far we've progressed in such a short amount of time. The average 55-year-old man or woman in the 1950s and '60s could be categorised as biologically elderly, with multiple (possibly undiagnosed) health conditions and probably only a decade or so left to live. In our new biological universe, a 55-year-old man or woman is just as likely to be planning a multi-day trip in the mountains and enjoying a performance spectrum previously only enjoyed by professional athletes. It's an amazing and humbling progression.

However, this level of fitness and training carries a small hypothetical risk, or at least a question mark. The experts are lavish with their praise for the physical and cognitive benefits that will accrue to you if you exercise moderately – these benefits go way beyond any medicine or drug ever invented. But cross the threshold into immoderation and the picture becomes a little more conflicted. For example, some of us may be embedding some cardiovascular remodelling, but even that may turn out to be protective in itself. The inevitable consequence of a current lack of clear conclusions and explanations, which will eventually flow from detailed longitudinal studies, means that in this moment we're all forced to make personal risk assessments about how we live and ride. We've made a point of flagging up where we think certain individuals should take extra clinical pre-emptive steps to ensure risks are reduced when they undertake strenuous training. For the rest of us, I suggest an attitude of informed, optimistic pragmatism in the face of a relentless flow of poorly researched populist tabloid articles on the risks that we may hypothetically face by exercising too hard when we're 'too old'. Maybe the best riposte for now is the suitably laconic comment by a cardiologist on the anomalous risks we face: 'So where are all the bodies?'

One of the unexpected twists in this book, however, was the apparent sex divergence in terms of cardiac risk. Female midlife athletes just don't seem to be exposed to the same exercise dose-related risk as men – the research to date seems very clear. Female athletes can exercise as hard as they like, as often as they like and will receive ever-increasing benefits with little risk or complication. But what's protecting them? Is just one hormone, oestrogen, affording all this protection on its own, or are there other lifestyle factors involved? Dr Parry-Williams took off her stethoscope for a moment, to hypothesize in a broader way about how men and women process stress, and the role of our sympathetic and parasympathetic nervous systems. Bluntly – are men predisposed to spend more of their lives in a fight or flight state relative to women? And if so, at what cost? And more importantly, what positive steps could men take to effect real change in their outlook and stress burden? Chapter 8, on mindful cycling, is an invitation for us all to live a little better as people as well as athletes, but I cannot help thinking that men, in general, probably have a little more homework to do here. I suspect, very strongly, that Dr Parry-Williams is onto something, and this makes this last chapter the most important in this book, in my opinion.

I'm going to leave you with a few thoughts until we meet again. The first is to remember that endurance cycling – the kind most of us do, most of the time – is aerobic or oxidative. The coaches and the team doctors agree that the biggest difference between amateurs and professionals is how close we, as amateurs, train to our theoretical red line, relative to the pros. I think this is partly borne out of the distracting obsession with FTP, power measurement and indoor cycling. To be clear: a high 20-minute FTP will not get you through a day in the mountains and a lack of experience actually riding your bike outside in the real world will not help you descend an Alpine pass quickly and safely. I see it all the time with our new clients. They misguidedly believe they must start their cycling journey fixated on their power numbers – trying to move into the penthouse before the foundations have been laid.

It's a big mistake from which we can all learn. Working on building our oxidative energy system is our equivalent of a sustainable solar or wave-power green energy source. In contrast, relying on anaerobic/lactate systems is like embedding a dependence on structurally unsustainable and uneconomic fuel sources, such as coal and nuclear. Not cool anymore.

And secondly, you're not a robot or a machine. You're a complex, intelligent and emotional person. Tuning your engine in the long term necessarily means creating a physical and emotional equilibrium. These are the newest ideas from progressive thinkers, coaches and sports physiologists like John Kiely, who are convinced that our mental state is a major contributor to training and adaption outcomes. I'm convinced that the forward thinking of people such as John Kiely and Dr Parry-Williams is where so much of the good work will come in making midlife cyclists even faster and healthier in the future.

Ironically, during the writing of this book, I developed some errant heart rhythms, just as I was writing chapter 3, 'Will I die?'. After ignoring the symptoms for a week or so I called my friend, Dr Mandeville, during a particularly intrusive episode. Dr Mandeville asked me a series of questions and calmly reassured me that I didn't need to head to A&E at that precise moment but the diagnostics that followed with my GP and hospital were not at all reassuring – there was something fundamental amiss. Further tests with Dr Stephens bought a clearer picture. I was advised to make changes to my life – reduce stress, reduce alcohol, slow down a little and look after myself more. But I was also advised that I could and should keep exercising and riding my bike. Which was, of course, thrilling news. Now I still ride hard on occasion, but I never ride 10/10ths – that's my choice. I don't drink alcohol because the effects on heart rhythms are now well known and uncontested. I'm more aware of my ANS and try to spend some time every day consciously invoking a parasympathetic state. I'm doing everything I can. I may well need a pacemaker in the future and that's also OK because I'll still be able to train and ride. I'll follow the advice of my doctors when that day comes. I never had to think of any of these things when I was racing in my 20s, 30s and 40s, but now I'm in my late 50s I do. I can't make myself perpetually young, but I can make sure that my wisdom and common sense increases to meet the challenges of maintaining health, speed and strength.

So unshackle yourself from your stationary trainer and your power meter. Go out into nature on your bike and take a few breaths. Remember that trying to make old people young again is the ultimate fool's errand. But trying to make old people fast is fun, life-affirming and almost certainly good for us.

Until next time.

Phil

MIDLIFE CYCLISTS: CASE STUDIES

A friend of mine is a veteran triathlete, as well as being a veteran GP and sports physician in Wisconsin, in the US. He gave me some of the best advice, and we remember it almost every day at Cyclefit. 'You can't learn everything all at once, it is simply impossible. But you can learn from your clients one condition at a time.' It was the best advice because it took all the pressure off us to be 'experts' who were meant to know everything about everyone's cycling injuries all the time.

Over the years we've been incredibly fortunate to be able to learn from our clients one issue at a time. Many clients go on to become experts in their own injury and condition, as a by-product of their unique experience and the research that they do around the subject. We've also had the opportunity to work with many dedicated and talented clinicians, consultants and physical therapists.

The first person we ever worked closely with was polymath physio Graham Anderson, 20 years ago. We were dumbfounded when the great man himself decided to devote a full morning a week, for well over a year, working alongside us with our clients. It gave us an appreciation for a multidisciplinary approach to both client care and communal learning. An early breakthrough came with a former elite racer called Ethan, who confounded us in our fitting studio. He felt profoundly low in power everywhere but especially on one side. We weren't at all happy and referred him to Graham. Graham was even less happy when he took a femoral pulse and referred him straight to a cardiologist, who operated the next day to replace a torn aorta. This was an unusual case of course,

265

but it was consistent with everyone trying to manage the problem, which isn't necessarily the same as trying to own it.

Ethan went through convalescence and rehab with Graham and then full circle back to us to check his biomechanics. He's still training and riding a couple of decades later. Very occasionally we get clients who have a similar issue and put them in touch with Ethan. The learning circle closes once again.

All of the case studies in this book are both clients and friends. All of them are back riding at a good level and not inhibited by the problems that they had. We've learned from our clients, and also our own personal experience, that sometimes you feel like you're in a maze with no route out. That's almost never the case – you just need to find the right guide, or two.

Case study I – atrial fibrillation (AF)

I have ridden with Kevin for decades – we've climbed mountains, competed in one-day events and raced literally hundreds of criteriums together as close teammates. Kevin is also a Cyclefit client and I therefore know his biomechanics almost as well as I know my own. Kevin was engaged with his AF on a clinical level but strangely not outwardly stressed by it. Entirely pragmatic, rational and, whenever I was with him, admirably calm. Which, as anyone who has ever raced with Kev will tell you, isn't always the case! Ahem!

I felt for Kevin because the lag from first symptoms to his ablation felt like a long time. Kevin's AF and treatment coincided with the very recent awareness that AF may be more prevalent for midlife male athletes. I think Kevin's own insight that alcohol was a contributory factor in bringing on an attack of AF is fascinating and now well known. But even more interesting is that not one clinician in his whole treatment path flagged it up. Kevin still rides all the time, but doesn't compete. He says: 'I started riding as a club junior aged 14. As an adult, I always used my bike for commuting and recreational riding, and then I started racing criteriums in my 40s. The earliest signs of AF came in my mid-50s, and showed as an elevated heart rate after strenuous riding, which would persist for 5–10 minutes after getting off the bike. The elevated heart rate would reach around 220bpm. It was very shallow and inefficient but not distressing. My normal max at that time was around 185bpm and resting 50bpm.

'Over a period of about four years the symptoms gradually increased in length and frequency and would also begin to occur when not exercising. By this stage, the AF would also impair my performance on the bike. Initially my AF was sporadic, therefore difficult to capture and diagnose. One morning I woke sweating with a heart rate of around 220bpm so I went to A&E. By the time I was seen by a doctor, my heart rate was back to normal and so I was sent home.

'With increasing AF I was initially given a 24-hour heart rate monitor, which didn't capture the AF. After six months I was given a seven-day heart rate monitor, and by this stage I was able to induce AF through strenuous effort and so ensure the AF was recorded and diagnosed.

'I was referred for an ablation. From diagnosis to treatment was around nine months. My ablation was successful first time. The prognosis was that the AF wouldn't return but that I might experience occasional short irregular heartbeats, which I do.

'I was advised not to ride or exercise strenuously again. I have ignored this advice with no ill effects. However, I now have a disinclination to push too hard and I no longer race. Also, my resting heart rate has increased by around 15bpm and my max has decreased by the same. I was advised this is in part due to the ablation and also ageing.

'I was given no advice regarding diet or alcohol. However, during the latter stages of my AF I recognised a correlation between alcohol consumption and the occurrence of AF, usually when riding the next day.'

Case study II – heart attack, Dr David Hulse

We got a text from Dave from St George's hospital late in the evening, saying that he had suffered a heart attack. Dave is a very close and valued friend – we've ridden, worked with and learned from Dave for 15 years. Four months after his heart attack we're riding with him in Richmond Park celebrating his 50th birthday and he's riding strongly at the head of the pack.

Dave's case study is interesting for many reasons. Firstly, because he's a doctor himself, so he brings his own insight into his symptoms and treatment. Secondly, his remarkable recovery (and survival) is almost certainly due to him being a fit cyclist for so many years. It's a positive message for all of us.

And lastly, his curiosity and commitment to look outside of the purely physical, for his own contributory factors, for lessons for living a better life. Dr Dave has become the riding personification of the mindful cyclist.

As an aside, Dave sent us notes and thoughts all the way through his treatment and recovery. He's the epitome of a great doctor – engaged, fascinated, modest and above all very decent. Great to have you back, Doc.

He says: 'Mortality greets us in many guises. I was an ostensibly fit 49-year-old husband and father, with two young children, and a lifelong cyclist. It had been a long and all-consuming February day, including an hour of strength training in the gym, and I was packing for an early morning flight. The onset was sudden – throat, jaw and upper-chest pain, quite unlike the textbook descriptions, but severe and unusual enough to warrant an ambulance. The ECG showed minor ischaemia, but blood tests confirmed myocardial injury – a heart attack. The questions were immediate: What happened? Why me? Why now? And what on earth did the future hold? An angiogram confirmed some impressive narrowings of my coronary arteries. A couple of days later, I drifted off to sleep at the hands of the anaesthetist and woke up hours later having undergone open heart bypass surgery. The emotions were raw in the early days. Before surgery I had been the youngest in a room of fellow inmates, all awaiting potentially life-changing and life-threatening procedures. On the day I left hospital I sought out John, who'd had his more major procedure the day after mine. He was OK. I held his hand, we wished each other well, and when I got back to my room the emotion flooded out.

'Cardiac rehabilitation began immediately, walking daily. The first was a lap of my local park. I was slow, but the fresh air was motivating. I slept that afternoon, exhausted but looking forward. The duration and distance were slowly increased over the following weeks. We had decided to escape the city for rural recuperation in Scotland, where I had spent youthful days cycling mile upon mile in scenery. Those days suddenly felt less distant. Flat became undulating; slow became moderate; and grey winter replaced by emergent spring. Six weeks after surgery marked a significant leap forward. I was allowed back on my road bike. The significance of that first hour ride cannot be overstated. My instructions were to limit my heart rate to 125bpm, and not to stress my healing sternum by putting weight through the bars. Betablockers were an interesting "limiter", and felt as though I had a diesel engine minus the turbocharger. The headspace of those rides was transforming and gave my uncertainties and anxieties much-needed perspective. The green shoots and birdsong of spring were a metaphor. My fitness and strength progressively improved and, now four months post-surgery and having turned 50, I feel almost "normal" and I'm discovering the answers to the "why?". We all carry genetic baggage, and mine contained a family history of cardiovascular disease that surely I could overcome with lifestyle. Except that I was no longer the 30-something veteran of multiple L'Étapes. I was a father, I had a career that required mental energy and emotion, and I was mortal, as we all are. Stress in all its forms – lifestyle and family, sport and training, good and bad – is cumulative. We may compartmentalise it based on source, but it can have the same physiological effects. Our genes and our psychology determine the degree of potential harm. Cycling is a wonderful, mindful release but, in common with all sporting endeavour, is also a source of stress that must be respected and balanced.'

Case study III – overtraining syndrome (OTS)

Matt has been a client and friend and riding partner for over 20 years. Which means that when he suffered his very serious bout of OTS, he was, somewhat embarrassingly, my client. I recall talking to him about his training around that time and being faintly disquieted by the combination of volume and intensity. I seem to remember trying to caution him about doing too much and not overcooking it. A few things to say about Matt's case. Firstly I'm much less circumspect now about how I express my advice in this regard whenever I suspect a client is doing too much. Secondly, I think we learned, alongside Matt, just how serious overtraining syndrome is and can be. It has the potential to be a very serious illness, with potentially profound consequences. And lastly, Matt is an extremely intelligent and also highly motivated individual – he was loving his riding and relishing the challenge. Not always the best recipe for moderation! Matt and I ride often together these days and I would say that he's totally recovered – he's strong and well-conditioned, but probably also more minded now to look at the holistic aspects of his life from his brush with OTS.

He says: 'It was the autumn of 2003, and I had never heard of OTS. I had, however, decided to do the L'Étape du Tour the following year, having previously done it in 2000. Having semi-retired the previous year, I figured I'd have the time to really push myself, and to see, for the first time, how good I could be. So, I started training…hard! That meant logging 500km per week or more, and resorting to spinning classes, sometimes 3 in a row, when it rained. Not surprisingly, I started improving. Then, early in the spring, I came down with a cold. No big deal, I figured, so I just kept riding, and I continued to improve. The virus lingered, and a few weeks later, I started having quite bad headaches. After a few weeks, I decided to see a doctor. I was poked, prodded, and scanned, but no cause was found. I decided to "tough it out", and kept training.

'A couple of weeks before the L'Étape, I was still feeling lousy, and noticed my performance dipping, suddenly and severely. I figured I needed a rest, so I took a few days off before heading by car to France. Once on the road, things got worse. I noticed that my resting heart rate was above 100bpm, and it went to 140 every time I stood up. I didn't sleep at all in the hotel, because of a terrible headache and the sound of my heart banging in my ears.

'On the night before the L'Étape, I knew something was really wrong, and decided not to do the event. But the following morning, one of my friends convinced me to at least start the ride, knowing that I could always bail out. In a final case of mind over matter, I completed the L'Étape, and headed home.

'By the time I arrived back in London, I'd been sleepless for four consecutive nights, my resting heart rate was 110bpm, and I was dizzy every time I stood up. I went back to my GP and once again began the process of trying to figure out what was going on. After several MRIs, a PET scan and a visit to the cardiologist, I was no closer to an answer. Finally, doing my own research on the internet, I discovered overtraining syndrome, otherwise known as unexplained underperformance syndrome. The symptoms seemed to match, and I discovered that Dr Richard Budgett, a physician working with the UK Olympic Team, was one of the foremost experts in the field.

'He saw me the following week, confirmed the diagnosis, and told me that I had one of the worst cases he'd ever seen. He recommended almost total rest, lots of sleep, and said not to allow my heart rate to exceed 100, even when walking. He said that the symptoms would gradually improve over the course of weeks and months, and they did. It took about six months to return to a semblance of normality.

'It was a terrifying experience, and I'm far more careful now. I still train hard, but when I'm ill I take it easy. The headaches and dizziness were symptoms I should have taken more seriously and then the dip in performance should have been a dead giveaway. My advice to anyone reading this is to watch for the signs. This isn't something you want to deal with.'

Case study IV – Dr Nigel Stephens

I am pleased that Nigel's case study made it into *The Midlife Cyclist*. At the time of writing all hospitals are struggling with a dangerous second wave of Covid-19, and Nigel's is no exception, but he selflessly gave his time to put together this case study in his coffee break.

I have known Nigel for many years, as a client, friend, treating cardiologist; we even raced together many years ago. Sessions with Nigel are always fantastic fun. It is just great to be in a room with someone so committed and erudite on all aspects of human physiology and performance.

I really felt for him with this crash (he has had others). The timing was just bloody awful. I spoke to him a week or so before the crash and he was gently very optimistic about his chances at the World's. And therefore, so was I. It was both a huge injury but also a massive psychological blow.

He limped into my studio on a quiet Saturday in October 2017. His outer frailty disappeared once he got kitted up and carefully mounted the jig, which I had set up in his race-bike position. You could see how much it meant to him to be back in racekit and clipped-in and pedalling. A typical bikeracer.

We worked closely over the next six weeks or so. I was concerned to make recovering/maintaining his normal pedalling function my priority; as well as unloading and therefore protecting the left hip structure. I knew I could rely on Nigel's unrivalled work ethic to recover and ameliorate the worst effects of atrophy and muscle function – I just had to give him a safe environment to work in.

It was a hugely satisfying and fascinating project from every perspective. Nigel had a great team, aside from us – the surgery and alignment was flawless, Alex Fugallo and Nigel's own treating phsyio. It was an object lesson in what is achievable when all the dots are correctly joined to give a great outcome.

He says: 'There are many lessons that could and should be learned from my unfortunate accident in the autumn of 2017. A quintessential mix of quite awful timing followed by a connective chain of good fortune.

'It was one of my last training rides before I was due to fly out to Los Angeles for the World Track Championships – I was in the form of my life. Should I have been out in the Hertfordshire lanes on a damp morning, in a group, only hours before an event that forms the cornerstone of my riding ambition? It is a good question and hindsight is always perfect. But it was a freak one in a thousand crash with unexpectedly dramatic repercussions.

'I lost the back wheel fast on an off-camber curve and knew rapidly after striking the road that it was a serious crash and injury. As a doctor (heart not bones), I was almost sure that I had suffered a very serious fracture of the left hip – I suddenly had one leg shorter than the other and the left leg was externally rotated. On that basis I had to resist my clubmates' well-intended entreaties to get back on my bike and ride (every racer's default setting). It was a very serious injury and not to be trifled with.

'At that precise moment a 4 × 4 vehicle turned up, who just happened to be on a remote recovery training exercise. The good fortune wheel has started to turn.

'After arriving at UCL Hospital in London, the bizarre trauma/pain-perception equation has flipped from partially anaesthetised to thoroughly uncomfortable, scream-out-loud painful.

'I am in surgery very quickly and the nature of the break (intertrochanteric fracture) has meant that surgery is likely to be largely successful, with a stronger repair. I have a large titanium shaft pushed into the femur, which is bolted at the top to the neck of the femur. The one-year mortality on such surgery is actually quite high at 25%; but in mitigation the most common cases are fragility fractures in elderly patients.

'I am discharged after only 18 hours by fulfilling the discharge phsyio criteria of climbing a flight of stairs. It is unquestionably premature (and maybe a record), but the hours and days post major surgery are precious in terms of recapturing mobility quickly. Muscle atrophy and a loss of neuromuscular connection and function occurs with brutal rapidity. I am working with a physio within 48 hours to gently encourage functional movements to help retain and restore neuromuscular movement patterns with respect to the leg in relation to pelvis. This is crucial from both a physiological but also psychological perspective.

'I walk on crutches into Phil's studio in Cyclefit, only 10 days after the crash. Racing kit and shoes on and I am under the microscope with my biomechanics and pedalling function under close scrutiny. The analysis shows that the injured side is actually working very poorly, and my right side is dramatically compensating by being overactive on the recovery phase (upstroke). If this is allowed to continue it could hamper my recovery in potentially three ways:

1   The left side will not be encouraged to load properly because it is being supported by the right side
2   The right side could become overactive and injured (especially hip flexors)
3   My normal pedalling motor-patterning will be eroded and difficult to recover.

I was not aware of any of this, by the way. The body makes its own adaptations.

'Phil's unpopular and drastic advice was to build a dedicated rehab position, to both offload the hip but also ensure that the left leg could not be assisted at all by the right leg.

His recommendation (which I followed to the letter) was:

- All riding for the rehab duration would be completed on flat pedals and not clipped in.
- 172.5mm cranks would be replaced by 160mm (to open the hip at the top of the pedal stroke).
- I was to use flat bars, short stem and raised bar position – also to keep hip open at the top of the pedal stroke.

I alternated seeing my physio, Phil and osteopath, Alex Fugallo, for the next few weeks. No possible stone was left unturned.

'By week 8 post surgery I was able to do 100km with my clubmates on my 'rehab bike' without pain or discernible loss of pace.

'Twelve weeks post-surgery I rode in my first track race (against Phil's advice). Lightning rarely strikes twice.

'And I now am now back racing at full strength and full function. If anything, I seem to be more powerful on my left side measured on a Dura–Ace power meter.

'What lessons are there to take away? The crash was hard and the injury serious. After that, my diagnosis was rapid and correct. My surgery was very well executed and appropriate. My rehab started in my mind the moment I woke up, and followed a path supported by professionals to its conclusion, in full strength and function. My role was to work hard and be compliant. Solicit good advice and then both believe it and take it.'

REFERENCES

Introduction and Prologue
Caspari, R., 2012, 'The Evolution of Grandparents', *Scientific American*, https://www.scientifi-camerican.com/article/the-evolution-of-grandparents-2012-12-07/

Chapter 1 – The Ageing Cyclist
Werner, C. et al., 2019, 'Differential effects of endurance, interval, and resistance training on telomerase activity and telomere length in a randomized, controlled study', *European Heart Journal*, https://academic.oup.com/eurheartj/article/40/1/34/5193508

Rogers, M.A., 1990, 'Decline in VO$_2$max with aging in master athletes and sedentary men', *Journal of Applied Physiology*, https://www.ncbi.nlm.nih.gov/pubmed/2361923

Harvard Women's Health Watch, 2015, 'Vigorous exercise may counter cognitive decline in early Alzheimer's', https://www.health.harvard.edu/mind-and-mood/vigorous-exercise-may-counter-cognitive-decline-in-early-alzheimers

Chapter 3 – Will I Die?
O'Keefe, J.H., et al. 2012, *Potential Adverse Cardiovascular Effects From Excessive Endurance Exercise* - https://www.ncbi.nlm.nih.gov/pmc/articles/PMC3538475/

Morris J.N., et al. 1953, *Lancet*, 'Coronary heart-disease and physical activity of work'.

Merghani A., et al. 2017, *Circulation*, 'Prevalence of Subclinical Coronary Artery Disease in Masters Endurance Athletes With a Low Atherosclerotic Risk Profile', https://pubmed.ncbi.nlm.nih.gov/28465287/

Baker, P., et al. 2019, *International Journal of Cardiology, Heart and Vasculature*, 'Exercise-induced cardiac troponin elevation: An update on the evidence, mechanism and implications', https://www.ncbi.nlm.nih.gov/pmc/articles/PMC6437282/

Koopman, F. A., et al. 2017, *Journal of Internal Medicine*, 'Balancing the autonomic nervous system to reduce inflammation in rheumatoid arthritis', https://pubmed.ncbi.nlm.nih.gov/28547815/

Machhada, A., et al. 2016, 'Vagal Tone and Exercise Capacity', UCL Centre for Cardiovascular and Metabolic Neuroscience, https://www.researchgate.net/publication/309488451_Vagal_tone_and_exercise_capacity

Chapter 4 – Midlife Performance
Kreher J. B., Schwartz J. B., 2012, 'Overtraining syndrome: a practical guide', *Sports Health*, https://pubmed.ncbi.nlm.nih.gov/23016079/

Chapter 8 – The Mindful Cyclist
Kiley J., 2018, *Sports Medicine, Periodization Theory: Confronting an Inconvenient Truth*, https://pubmed.ncbi.nlm.nih.gov/29189930/

Meier P. and Seitz H. K., 2008, *Current Opinion in Clinical Nutrition and Metabolic Care, Age, alcohol metabolism and liver disease*

ACKNOWLEDGEMENTS

I have learned that books are difficult to bring to life on your own. This book would not have happened without so many people's selfless input and wisdom. I am fortunate to have so many to thank. To mention a few:

First to Cyclefit co-founder, Julian Wall – we learnt together over 20 years, one client at a time. We shared every mystery and epiphany. Not a journey anyone could or should make on their own.

Next to the consultants, coaches, and academics who are featured in *The Midlife Cyclist*. A notable few of you, I continually called upon at an unprecedented time – and still you remained endlessly gracious and generous.

Graham Anderson, Dr Jonathan Baker, Mr Tim Briggs, Kathryn Brown, Garth Fox, Alex Fugallo, Professor Philip Goulder, Dr Derek Harrington, Dr David Hulse, Dr Nicky Keay, John Kiely, Dr Justin Mandeville, Dr Ahmed Merghani, Dr Gemma Parry-Williams, Dr Audrius Simaitis and Dr Nigel Stephens.

To my friends: Peter, Robin and Tony for a bulwark of intelligence and honesty.

To my editors: Matthew Lowing and Sarah Skipper for their wisdom, friendship and guiding light.

My mother Fran, late father Geoff and sister Jackie.

And finally, to my own precious family: my wife, Donna, and daughter Scout, for everything that matters most.

Oh, and Raff, the dog, for lying on my feet under my desk for the entire 120,000 words.

Phil Cavell

'Thou shouldst not have been old till thou hadst been wise.'
King Lear, Shakespeare

INDEX

AUTHOR BIOGRAPHY

Phil is joint founder of the pioneering Cyclefit organisation – the first company in Europe dedicated to cycling analysis and biomechanics. Cyclefit has run worldwide education programmes as well as providing bike-fitting services to professional cycling teams and athletes.